TAKE BACK YOUR HEALTH

Learn how your diet impacts your health, both good and bad, so that you can then use food as medicine.

George Elder
www.takebackyrhealth.com

ISBN-13: 9798564726825

Cover design by: Art Painter
Library of Congress Control Number: 2018675309
Printed in the United States of America

PREFACE

This is my book about my discovery, review of research and transition to the Low Carb / Keto diet.

In my 30's I was diagnosed with hypertension. A surprising condition as I was marathon training and I believed I was eating well. This was followed by a number of tests and a heart X-Ray, but in the end the doctor said I had to go onto blood pressure (BP) medications. When I asked about other options, he laughed, so I found another doctor.

For 2 years I studied and adopted a Pritikin diet and continued a basic low fat diet for many years. Eventually, in my 50's, I began one BP medication which over time grew into a higher dose and then a second medication. By the age of 60 my cholesterol and triglycerides were rising and the doctor started talking about statin drugs.

One night my wife and I happened to watch a video about our western diet and I was astonished. Everything I thought I knew about healthy eating was turned on its head. Was healthy low fat a myth? Could this be real? Determined to investigate further, I began researching and reading voraciously. I visited local libraries brought home 3 or 4 books at a time and began to build up a reading list of everything that was referenced. I have now built up a personal library of over 200 books, most written by doctors who have personally experienced problems with standard dietary advice and this has led me to discover the way of eating outlined in this book.

With all the research I reviewed, the science began to stack up and I became better at identifying fake dietary advice. My wife and I switched to a Low Carb / High Fat (LCHF)/Keto diet and I started keeping notes, to help reinforce what I was learning. As the notes grew, it became my reference book. I then found other interested people wanted a smaller, simpler book.

The result is this book, based on all the books, stories, medical research reports, podcasts, YouTube videos, etc. that I have undertaken read and watched. It also documents our N=2 experience adopting this way of living over a 4 year period.

I am also the proud holder of a Diploma in Nutrition from "The Nutrition Institute" and a certificate in Sports Nutrition.

In an effort to minimise the possibility of "confirmation bias" I read widely, particularly authors who have gained a strong following over the years, but whom I find to have flawed dietary advice. I won't name them for obvious reasons but I frequently find their books in book sales and purchase them for the home library.

Because the field of nutrition research is developing fast, I find that books and papers first published more than a few years ago, often have statements or views that have been recently superseded or debunked by better and new research. This is particularly true of statements about the dangers of saturated fat (SFA). It is only in August 2020 that the American College of Cardiology published their paper stating: *"Whole-fat dairy, unprocessed meat, and dark chocolate are SFA-rich foods with a complex matrix that are not associated with increased risk of CVD. The totality of available evidence does not support further limiting the intake of such foods"*.

This continuing mountain of updated of nutrition and diet

research means that what you understand may need to be updated. However not all research is truthful.

I manage a website where I publish blogs and information as I gain more understanding of this fascinating field of knowledge. This is available for free at https://www.takebackyrhealth.com. Where you can read free articles and where I have provided a number of resources for readers. The website highlights publications I have found to be excellent, that you may enjoy reading. There are meal plans, food tables, guides plus other resources for people choosing to make this dietary change.

Happy reading.   https://www.takebackyrhealth.com

CONTENTS

INTRODUCTION

When I discovered that my knowledge about diets and nutrition was almost all rubbish, I was motivated to search through research, nutrition and diet guidance to seek out quality and true information. I was appalled at the misinformation and dogma that dominates this field. I was also shocked at the poor quality of information provided to people about diet and health. I reviewed research and began making notes to explain it to friends and family.

I discovered that older people with higher cholesterol levels live longer, that lower salt is bad for you, that saturated fat is good for you, wholegrains are not really very healthy, and sugar substitutes should be avoided, amongst other things.

So, here is a simple readable summary of what I now believe to be important information that everyone should know, to take back their health, and maybe lose weight as well. I have now lived this way for 4 years and although I am now 72, I am healthier, stronger and in better shape than the last 30 years.

First, I must include a disclaimer. <u>This is NOT medical advice. I am not a health professional, this is merely documenting what I have come to believe from my personal journey of research reviews and my personal results. Prior to making any changes to your diet or lifestyle, you should seek professional medical</u>

<u>advice from a registered health professional.</u>

You will likely have learned that wholegrains are healthy, that high cholesterol indicates increased risk of heart attacks, that more fiber improves gut health, that fruit is good for you and saturated fat is bad. From my reviews of research I have discovered that these claims are, more often, NOT true. You might be shocked, so I will keep it all quite brief but give you enough information to undertake your own research. I have included some links to relevant published research.

I hear on podcasts and read doctors claims that they don't learn about nutrition in depth and, so it is understandable that they may not ask about or give advice about eating healthy. Sometimes due to work pressures, they struggle to keep up to date with current research and findings. I see published articles by nutritionists that are in conflict with the latest research findings, suggesting that they may be advising their clients based on out-of-date information. Many professionals still think that saturated fat is to be avoided and that your LDL cholesterol level is a good indicator of your risk of a heart attack despite the latest robust research.

In many countries and clinics, a doctor, dietitian or nutritionist is constrained by the organization they work in, or the 'standard of care' for the region and can be censured for advising anything different. When I asked a local doctor, in New Zealand, about a low carbohydrate diet, he answered that even if he thought it was the best option, he was not able to recommend it due to the rules he had to operate within. If you would like to follow up on this, search for the stories surrounding Professor Tim Noakes in South Africa, or Dr Gary Fettke from Australia and their censure for giving diet advice contrary to standard practise.

The field of nutrition research is changing quite rapidly as a result of new studies where we learn even more about how the human body functions. Just a few years ago doctors routinely treated stomach ulcers with surgical intervention, whereas we now know that the H. pylori infections causing this can usually be treated with antibiotics. Today we still have nutritionists who believe the low fat / high carb diet is healthy for everyone despite the obesity epidemic and all the evidence that many people get sick on this diet.

In the USA many doctors and clinicians are monitored by their employer and sponsors to ensure that they are prescribing the 'standard of care' level drugs and treatment. This is apparently done by reviewing patient notes, to ensure best possible revenue for the organisation and less possibility of any liability. However, this also means that clinicians have less discretion to make patient specific decisions and it appears this may be having a demoralising impact on their work satisfaction.

Most people have no idea that much of the plant-based diet messaging originates from religious beliefs and ideology, designed to demonize animal-based food without good scientific basis. For example, The Seventh Day Adventist Church, founders of vegetarianism, have on their website many documents about the evils of eating meat which they consider unclean. The American College of Lifestyle Medicine, Doctors for Nutrition, campaigns such as 10,000 toes, the CHIP program are active elements supported by this group plus they promote plant-based diets which they consider superior, with certification, through institutions to doctors and nutritionists.

Much medical and nutrition research is funded by drug manufacturers and food companies, who are seeking to convince you to eat their food or use their drugs. Unfortunately, if the research does not support their business plans, they don't want people to know, so negative results are sometimes not published or ignored. One major report (Minnesota Coronary Experiment, 1968-1973) was not published for 16 years, because it didn't come out the way they expected.

As an example of bias, in a recent review of 60 articles about whether sugar plays a role in obesity, 34 showed a direct link, but 26 recorded no association, but when looked at in more detail it was found that all of the 26 and 1 of the 34 were funded by the Sugar sweetened beverage industry. To follow up, take a look here: https://www.medscape.com/viewarticle/871167

A warning to those conducting their own research:

You may discover that many sources are quite biased in the information they provide and as a result you will need to consult multiple sources to confirm accurate information.

For example UK Dr. Malcolm Kendrick is an ardent critic of statin drugs and has written 3 books on this subject with his latest titled "The Clot Thickens". If you search for him on Google you will find plenty of information, however if you search for him in Wikipedia, they seem to have never heard of him. Censorship in action!

A search in Google for good sources of protein can turn up a list of only plant protein sources. Only by more direct searches will you come up with the animal foods which actually have superior protein levels and bioavailability.

Searches for nutrient levels in many foods often neglect to mention the important issues of bio-availability and the impact of anti-nutrients. These can both significantly reduce available nutrients to the consumer.

You will only get the information the author wants you to believe even if it is wrong or missing important elements. Censorship is rife.

I am fully aware of these difficulties, and have tried to ensure that I have presented a complete and accurate picture.

WHAT A MESS OUR HEALTH IS IN

In the 19th century and very early 20th century, the leading cause of death was infectious diseases and complications from infections. Heart attacks were very rare, type 2 diabetes was rare, macular degeneration was not yet in text books and obesity was uncommon. Shortly after WW2 governments decided to establish eating guidelines. About the same time, some businesses found that they had surplus products that could, with further processing, be sold as cooking oils, farming scaled up to use big machinery and the US Government began subsidising some grain crops, which resulted in reduced cost of food, particularly grains and sugar.

Everything had changed but our bodies hadn't changed, so now we have a very different mix of food and our bodies are not yet adapted. The result is much higher levels of sugars, processed carbohydrates and industrial seed oils in the Western diet than previously existed. The impact is shown in poor overall health with skyrocketing levels of type 2 diabetes, fatty liver disease, macular degeneration, kidney disease, increased tooth decay, and massive increases in obese and overweight people. Recent research has linked obesity to a much higher risk of many cancers.

Top Causes of Death in USA, 1900 vs 2010

Source: USA Center for Disease Control

	1900	2010
Other	36%	25%
Pneumonia or Influenza	12%	2%
Tuberculosis	11%	0%
Gastrointestinal infections	8%	0%
Heart disease	8%	24%
Stroke	6%	5%
Kidney disease	5%	2%
Accidents	4%	5%
Cancer	4%	23%
Senility	3%	3%
Diptheria	2%	0%
Suicides	-	2%
Diabetes	-	3%
Airways diseases	-	6%

People are now eating huge amounts of sugar, lots of wheat and corn-based foods (grains), and consuming huge quantities of industrial seed oils. Statistics from 2018, show that less than 12% of USA citizens are metabolically healthy and for older people the numbers are even worse.

Eating guidelines were heavily directed by some questionable science from Dr Ancel Keys an American physiologist with a degree in fish physiology who developed the K-ration pack during WW2, and, through his persistence, he became involved in the development of published USA eating guidelines in the 1970's. From research and some world travel, he became convinced that eating saturated fat was the cause of heart disease and the avoidance of this has influenced most major diet recommendations since that time.

A British doctor and professor of nutrition at University of London, John Yudkin, argued that sugar was the main culprit but was heavily and publicly ridiculed by Keys.

John Yudkin's book "Pure White and Deadly" is a good read. Modern researchers studying Keys' data have found serious flaws with his work, such as ignoring data from his major study (The Seven Countries Study) that did not support his views. Twenty-two countries were actually studied but he cherry picked the data that supported his hypothesis.

Why haven't we switched back to traditional diets? Food businesses are making lots of money, food delivery systems are set up for this type of food, many health providers are doing well, drug companies are selling lots of drugs. Many 'experts' including university-based leaders and researchers have their careers based on these guidelines, and there seems to be an underlying fear of change and lack of willingness to admit that current guidelines could be wrong.

It is not surprising that food companies and drug companies are pushing products that make them the most profit. That is what they are in business to do and what their owners and investors expect. They are acting like the tobacco companies did a few years ago which knowingly created uncertainty about the health impact of smoking by recruiting 'apparent experts' to challenge any information that denigrated smoking. We have to recognize that for these food and drug companies, our health is not their first priority, therefore, we should judge any claims they make by this standard.

Statistics show that our society is getting sicker. It seems that if you want to get off this bad diet train, you have to do your own research and make your own decisions about changing. It may be that you have to go against the tide, and thumb your nose at big food business, drug companies and ignore all the advertising you see around you in order to take back your health.

Alphabet groups like the heart associations and diabetes associations should be helping us, but they also receive significant funding by the same big businesses, so could be seriously conflicted and we need to carefully check the advice they provide. Experts recruited to create and review diet guidelines are usually conflicted by association and funding from big business.

Although we are starting to see some small changes, in general their advice often does not follow the latest health research conclusions. For example, some diabetes associations have websites recommending lots of carbohydrates for a type 2 diabetic diet. In Australia and New Zealand, take a critical look at the products which get a heart tick on the packet and draw your own conclusions.

If you choose to take back your health, you also have to be able to withstand the pressure of family and friends who have been bombarded for years with official diet guidelines, and now fully believe them. Most people's nutrition knowledge comes from friends, family, food packaging or media and magazine articles designed to sell products and influence, rather than to educate.

You might be told:

- that breakfast is the most important meal of the day,

- that saturated fat is unhealthy,

- that you need to eat carbohydrates to provide glucose to fuel your brain,

- that meat consumption will cause cancer,

- that cholesterol is bad and you may need to take drugs to lower this,

- that low salt is healthy.

- that cow burps cause climate change pollution that is worse than pollution from global transport.

From the latest science, it is now understood that these and many other beliefs are NOT true.

It is important to realise that the published official diet guidelines such as the USA 'food pyramid' and the UK 'food plate' are only applicable to metabolically healthy people. This means only about 20%, or less, of these populations.

Perhaps the best description of what is happening comes from Louise Stephen in her book 'Eating Ourselves Sick'. She contends that there is lots of research going on but it is being filtered through a few organisations and institutions who are interested in preserving the status quo and who actively filter the results to ensure you only get to see or read what they want you to see.

These organisations also work to actively counter any results that disagree with their view. This means that you must read outside mainstream channels to find out what is really being discovered.

Perhaps this is why UK Dr. Malcolm Kendrick is "missing" from Wikipedia.

A good resource to understand the history of diet guidelines and the impact of historical influences, is the link I have put to Belinda Fettke on YouTube, in the further learning pages, at the end of this book.

Also shown here: https://youtu.be/NEFvoyTMxVg

HOW DOES YOUR BODY WORK?

In order to understand what is right and what is wrong, let's take a simple look at how the human body works and we will begin to see why the official dietary guidelines are so out of step. Keep in mind that everyone is unique, so that there are some people out there who are slim and able to tolerate the official dietary recommendations, while there are others who appear to put weight on just by looking at food.

Let's start with food and nutrition. There are three macronutrients that we eat, Protein, Fat and Carbohydrates plus Fiber. Let's look at each of these to understand what happens when we eat them.

Protein

You must eat protein as it is used by your body for growth and repair. Without protein you get very sick. This is so important that we each have a protein appetite which helps control how much protein we eat. If your protein appetite is not satisfied, you will continue to feel hungry until it is satisfied.

At an absolute minimum, you need about 0.8 to 1.5 grams of protein every day, for every kilogram of body weight depending on your age and level of activity. Unfortunately, the foods we are eating more of today, are often 'Ultra processed' which reduces fiber, and depletes nutrients, resulting in low levels of protein but high energy levels.

If you are older, or very active, you will need more protein, up to 3 grams per kilogram of body weight. Eating a higher protein diet can reset your body's weight setpoint to a lower level. This is the weight level that the body is trying to maintain. Never reduce calories from protein while trying to achieve a calorie deficit, if anything you should increase protein.

A number of doctors advocating a high protein diet claim that you should eat at least 30 grams of protein in your first meal each day to kick-start muscle growth.

Proteins are made up of a number of amino acids. Your body separates these out and uses them for different processes. For example: tryptophan is one of the essential proteins (essential means that you must get it from your diet) and is used to manufacture serotonin (the happiness hormone) inside your body. Low tryptophan equals low serotonin.

Animal-based foods are a very good source of protein particularly as animal-based proteins provide a full complement of the essential amino acids needed.

Plants can provide protein, particularly soy. But on a plant-based diet, you need to carefully match the plant sources to ensure that the essential amino acids, missing from one source, are supplied by a complementary source. For example, eating rice with beans will supply a full set of essential amino acids.

While there are statements made about too much protein having a detrimental impact on kidneys, it appears this is only a problem for people with kidney disease. It is thought by some that stone-age people could have eaten up to 40% of their food energy as protein.

Dr. Ted Naiman MD and William Shewfelt's book 'A P:E diet' has an emphasis on eating food with a higher level of protein and a lower level of energy. Their concern is that by eating more carbohydrates and/or fat, it is possible to consume more energy than can be used by your body and get less nutrition than needed. The impact of this is that the body signals the need for additional food seeking to get the required protein and nutrients, and, therefore, drives overeating. Their view is that a 1:1 ratio of protein to energy by grams is desirable, but the excessive availability of 'low protein' processed food today has severely changed this ratio leading to typical diseases of civilization.

There is a known condition that afflicted arctic explorers, in the early 20th century, called 'rabbit starvation', which occurred during periods of limited food, when the explorers ate only rabbits because they were available. Rabbits have very very little fat, and this lack of fat caused sickness due to excess production of ammonia. The same issue plagued Vilhjalmur Stefanssen during the first few weeks of his year-long demonstration of survival on an all-meat diet, because the initial diet provided by the hospital, failed to include sufficient fat.

It seems that there is an upper limit to protein for humans which is around 40% of your calories. Levels above this may overwhelm the liver's ability to convert nitrogen from protein into urea causing ammonia levels to increase leading to stress in the body. Vilhjalmur Stefanssen is quoted as saying that rabbit starvation in the arctic could kill a person more quickly than eating nothing.

Some body builders attempt to get to these higher levels but it takes a concerted effort coupled with protein supplements and cannot be achieved on a typical diet.

Fat

Our bodies run on fat which is converted into fatty acids in our body. It comes from both plant and animal foods. Our brains are mostly fat, fat keeps us warm and provides a huge store of energy to keep our bodies moving, breathing, pumping blood, digesting food, etc. It is stored all over the body and comes in a number of dietary forms. We will examine each of these because some are good for you and some are not as good. Fat is critical to our survival and, particularly, for brain growth in children.

It is estimated that the average person has at least 130,000 calories stored as fat. Because of this store, and with the right conditions, a person who is fat-adapted can function without additional food for a lengthy period surviving off this store. Fat-adapted means that their body can easily operate either with fat as fuel or with glucose, whichever is available. This is sometimes termed metabolically flexible.

Many of the minerals and nutrients that the body requires are only delivered within the fat in our diets, particularly animal fats, and although some believe that plants can supply many of these nutrients, most plant forms are much less bio-available (absorbable when consumed). Examples include Vitamin A, D, E and K2. This is very important because if you eat no fat with these vitamins, they pass directly through the body becoming unavailable to you.

There are 3 classifications of fat all based on the structure of the fat molecule:

Saturated fat (SAT)   - Very stable
Mono-unsaturated fat (MUFA) - Mildly unstable
Poly-unsaturated fat. (PUFA)   - Powerfully unstable

Saturated fat makes up 48% of the fats in human mother's breast milk although this can vary due to many factors.

The term "Saturated Fat" conjures up images of artery clogging muck. Unfortunately this image is completely wrong and the name relates only to the structure of the molecule. My suggestion of a better way to think of these fats is:

Stable Fat
Mildly Unstable Fat
Powerfully Unstable Fat

Carbohydrates

All carbohydrates are made from sugar. This is the only macronutrient that we can actually live healthily without because your liver can manufacture glucose from fat and protein as needed. Some traditional diets have few or almost zero carbohydrates. The traditional Inuit diet is a prime example. However, in about 1980 government guidelines recommended we eat a much higher level of carbohydrates than had been historically the case.

Most carbohydrates are immediately converted to glucose/sugar in the body, whether they come from sugar, bread, fruit, pasta, rice or vegetables. Your body stores glucose in the liver and the muscles as glycogen, with a very small amount (about 1 teaspoonful) held as blood sugar in the blood. Having glucose in the muscles puts it right where it is needed for emergency muscle action such as running for your life.

It is estimated that the average person has about 2,500 calories stored as glycogen.

Glucose is a key fuel for the body, but because you cannot store very much, if your body is running on glucose, you need to eat regularly such as every 3-4 hours. Just to repeat, carbohydrates are not essential, meaning that the lowest limit for them in a human is zero, because your liver will make any glucose you need from fats.

Your body cannot store much glucose (or glycogen), so should you have an excess, your body will convert this to fat and store it.

Your body operates on a concept of "Oxidative Priority" which means that certain food groups are prioritised over others for energy, (The Randle Cycle). Carbohydrates have a higher priority than fats which means that if you consume lots of carbohydrates plus fats in a single meal, the fats cannot be utilised until the carbohydrate level is lowered. The result is fats can get pushed into body storage because the excess carbohydrate is dominating the energy supply within your mitochondria.

This effect may be why research has found benefits for choosing to eat carbohydrates at the end of a meal.

There are some groups that claim the Inuit people's ability to survive and remain healthy with very little carbohydrate in the Arctic, is some sort of genetic adaption. However, this is contradicted by the fact that early European Arctic explorers living with the Inuit and eating traditional Inuit food were able to happily adopt their diet for years without any loss of health.

Common carbohydrates include sugar, grains, flour, bread, honey, cereals, potatoes, corn, beer, fruit juice, rice and high fructose corn syrup. Of course, all the products made with any of these ingredients contain significant amounts of carbohydrate. To get an idea of the different levels of sugar in some foods, I provide some examples: (tsp = teaspoon)

120 grams banana	5.7 tsp of sugar
150 grams boiled potato	9.1 tsp of sugar
80 grams sweet corn	4 tsp of sugar
60 grams raisins	10.3 tsp of sugar
120 grams strawberry	0.4 tsp of sugar
Wholemeal bread, small slice	3.0 tsp of sugar
80 grams broccoli	0.2 tsp of sugar

For help identifying the level of sugar in common food items see: https://phcuk.org/sugar/

Fiber

This is usually a carbohydrate but it is different because it is not readily absorbed by the body. Fiber helps slow down the absorption of the food energy and helps the body feel full.   Although some people believe adding dietary fiber is unnecessary for your diet, others believe that it is very important to add for your health.   As a result of reading and reviewing research, I have now come to believe that eating grains, fruit or vegetables to maintain your fiber intake is unnecessary.

I am reminded that breastfed babies get no additional dietary fiber and definitely have no difficulty pooping.

The vegetables with high fiber and producing the highest levels of short chain fatty acids (SCFA), the fermentable prebiotic that feeds your microbiome, belong to a group known as fructo-ogliosaccharides. This group includes bananas, onions, garlic, chicory root, leeks and Jerusalem artichoke. The next highest food for SCFA is collagen followed by chicken cartilage. Eating a variety of animals foods nose to tail provides protein, fats and fiber. A meal including ribs (for example) will provide all the fiber necessary along with plenty of other nutrients.

Beta-hydroxybutyrate the main ketone body produced as a result of adopting a ketogenic diet is also a short chain fatty acid (SCFA), and feeds the microbiome as a prebiotic.

Perhaps the most important point I have learned is to avoid fiber from grains as this apparently can be damaging to your intestines. I would suggest you do not need to chase fiber because it is in many foods we eat including fish, meat, fruits and vegetables.   When eating fruit ensure you eat the whole fruit, including fiber, as the fiber can reduce the impact of the insulin spike caused by the body responding to the incoming fructose.

Some primitive diets have very little fiber, but others have very high fiber levels. Insoluble fiber, like bran, will fill out stools, but soluble fiber is more beneficial for lowering insulin. Surprisingly, recent tests have busted another fiber myth by showing that reducing fiber in the diet can correct severe constipation. Checkout this link: https://www.ncbi.nlm.nih.gov/pmc/articles/ PMC3435786/ and prepare to be amazed.

The conclusion of the above study was: *"Idiopathic constipation and its associated symptoms can be effectively reduced by stopping or even lowering the intake of dietary fiber."* As the Australian Doctor Paul Mason said, *"adding dietary fiber to reduce constipation is like adding more cars to a freeway to reduce congestion, it makes no sense"*.

A low carbohydrate diet involves the reduction of grains, fruit and starchy vegetables and therefore removes a very high volume of the fiber that you have been used to eating. Both soluble and insoluble fiber plus the overall bulk of the stools are affected by this transition. As a result, the urge to poop is reduced and if you may fail to notice it. It is important that you try to get into a regular habit of anticipating the urge in the early days, because failing to notice means that the stools although smaller, can remain in the colon longer and, as a result, can become dry and hard making then uncomfortable to expel.

In time this resolves as, 1. You become more aware of the less urgent poop sensations, 2. Your intestine gradually shrinks from a stretched condition, from past fiber-filled large stools, which then improves motility. While this can be a little uncomfortable, the benefits of a lower fiber diet are many and your future health should improve as a result. This does mean that you should be hyper aware of the need-to-poop signal and not postpone the event as you can reduce your comfort as a result.

There is no negative impact of the smaller stools and I would not recommend supplementing additional fiber or medication to bulk up the stool in any way. There are many research papers going back some years showing that a lower fiber diet does NOT increase your risk for colon cancer and can ease common intestinal complications, despite these results being ignored by many agencies and medical specialists. This link is one example:

https://doi.org/10.1056/NEJM199901213400301

One of the most visible changes that I noticed after adopting a ketogenic diet is that I poop less often, occasionally missing a day and there is no discomfort or concern. Possibly because I missed the urge to go signal as described above. I have come to realise that I don't have constipation, I am just utilizing a greater portion of the food I ate, plus I am eating less fiber, resulting in a smaller poop size.

Some carbohydrates can have their 'fiber' level raised, and insulin impact reduced, by creating resistant starch. To do this, cook the carbohydrate (such as rice, oats, beans or potato) cool overnight in the refrigerator and then eat or reheat. This changes the chemistry of the starch in the food raising the resistant starch level by up to 3 times and reducing the glycaemic load.

Resistant starch, is not digested in the small intestine and, therefore, becomes available as food for the microbiome in the large intestine. In this way it functions as a prebiotic.

The process of cooking and cooling reduces the glycaemic load of the food thereby reducing its ability to rapidly spike insulin.

Foods with high levels of resistant starch:
  (Max grams per 100gms)
    Barley (16)
    Green banana flour   (68)
    Potato Starch, unheated (79)
    Hi-Maize / Corn starch (58)
    Casava starch (80)
    Cashews (12.9)

The following cooked and cooled foods:
    Rice (cooked and cooled) (5.4)
    Potato (boiled and cooled) (3.2)
    Potato (Boiled and frozen for 30 days) (12)
    Potato (Roasted and cooled) (19.2)
    Beans and lentils
    Oats

To maximise the benefit of this chemistry, you could cook a larger amount, cool and then use for later meals. This might be a method to reduce the impact of eating some rice while still minimising the glycaemic load impact of this and may help with transitioning to a rice free diet eventually.

I have found cauliflower rice will adequately replace the rice I previously ate in meals and can be purchased pre-prepared and frozen in supermarkets. Check the ingredients list to ensure that it only contains cauliflower.

YOUR METABOLISM

Humans have two primary (plus some smaller) energy systems, a fat-based system where the body runs on fatty acids, and a carbohydrate-based system where your body runs on glucose.

You have huge energy stores of fat, but only small energy stores of carbohydrate. These two systems operate side by side, but what you consume ultimately conditions your body to what it uses for fuel. A person who is described as 'metabolically flexible' is able to easily switch between the two primary systems.

Humans have a metabolic oxidation priority. What does this mean? When your body needs energy it selects from the top of this stack (shown overpage). Your body takes from the top in order and avoids (not completely) using anything below until the higher up items are mostly exhausted. Unfortunately, body fat is at the very bottom of the stack.

Here is the stack order for humans:

<u>Oxidation Priority Stack</u>

1. Alcohol

2. Ketones

3. Excess Protein

4. Blood Sugar (from Carbohydrates)

5. Glycogen (Glucose stored in liver or muscle)

6. Free Fatty Acids in blood

7. Body Fat.

In essence this means that if you ingest alcohol, all other metabolic processes are put on hold and if you want to use body fat for energy, all the other sources have to be depleted. A high carbohydrate diet loads up blood sugar followed by glycogen, thereby preventing your body from using dietary fat or accessing body fat. This also shows that if eating fat and carbohydrates together the fat cannot be utilised and will be stored. If the body is making ketones from fat, then these are oxidised for energy first.

The simple mechanism of a low-carbohydrate diet is revealed here whereby it minimizes 4 and 5, keeps excess carbs from being converted to fat plus allows the body to oxidize fatty acids then (at last) to use stored body fat.

If you eat more food than you can use immediately, your body stores the excess as body fat. Looking back at the Oxidative Priority Stack, excess of number 4 (Blood Glucose is stored as 5 (glycogen) and then 7 (Body Fat). Excess of 6 (Fatty acids in blood) is stored as 7 (Body fat). There is a hormone in the body called insulin that is released when you eat, and one of its jobs is to manage fat storage. Different foods stimulate insulin in different ways with refined carbohydrates creating the biggest spike in insulin levels and dietary fat having a very low impact. Insulin also manages the release of fat, so if insulin rises, use of body fat stops.

Human babies are born quite chubby and use their body fat to nourish their growth and brain development. Breastfed babies are often in what is known as a state of ketosis. This is where their body is using fat for brain growth and energy, both from breast milk and by the breakdown of their own body fat.

As the baby grows, the body learns to eat and use more carbohydrates. Your body will always use some fatty acids and glucose, but will prioritize glucose if it is available, switching to burning fat from your diet, or from body fat, when the glucose level drops. The body is a very smart mechanism, whereby it will save excess energy and store it as body fat, for use at a later time, particularly when there is limited food available. This mechanism ensures that you never run out of one of the two energy forms, which is essential to staying alive.

As you can see, we eat to provide energy, we use the energy as needed, and we store the excess as body fat to use later when food is not available. This model has worked very well for thousands of years when food was sometimes plentiful and sometimes scarce.

However, these days we are lucky that there are very few occasions when food is unavailable. In fact, we are (badly) advised to eat lots of small meals throughout the day and we have developed the concept of snacking, so that we are eating every few hours. In addition, we advise people to get their body working by eating breakfast immediately they get up in the morning. Modern breakfasts are often very carb heavy with cereals, breads and fruit juices. We have learned to fear running out of food and we go to great lengths to make sure this doesn't happen.

The current official recommendations to eat lots of carbohydrate daily can create quite an engineering challenge for your body, as the carbs are immediately converted to sugar/ glucose but too much sugar is toxic and so your body has to find somewhere to put all this glucose. More than about 1 teaspoon of sugar in the blood is toxic, and your body is designed to maintain this level by converting and storing the excess as fat. This continual high carbohydrate load also ensures that any dietary fat cannot be used immediately and therefore will be stored.

First your body will ensure that muscles are loaded with glycogen, then top up the liver and if there is still too much, it will convert glucose to fat and store it in fat cells. If fat cells become insulin resistant and refuse the glucose, then the body must still remove it from the blood so it forces it into the liver, eventually and over time, creating Non-Alcoholic Fatty Liver Disease. (NAFLD).

During World War II, Dr. Ancel Keys conducted some starvation research (The Minnesota Starvation Experiment) on 36 fit young men in the USA. Feeding them a low fat, mostly carbohydrate diet of only 1600 calories a day proved to be a disaster. They lost on average 15 pounds over half a year, became cold, hair fell out, they became emaciated, had suicidal thoughts, two had breakdowns and one ended up in an institution. At the end of the experiment, they ate huge amounts of food, all ending up much fatter than when they started. On a predominantly carbohydrate diet, when the level goes low, the body responds by generating extreme hunger signals.

As a direct and very telling comparison, in 1970's researchers Bistrian and Blackburn, at Harvard Medical School, prescribed a diet that reduced calories for thousands of patients to 650-800 calories per day. Called 'A Protein Sparing Modified Fast', the patients happily lost weight with zero ill effects, half losing 40 pounds or more. The difference was that this diet was heavy on meat and fish with almost zero carbohydrate. Unfortunately, the researchers discontinued this approach because they believed, at that time, that continuing a very low carbohydrate diet was unhealthy.

Dr. Keys disastrous experiment mirrors the standard recommendations that are given to people who need to lose weight, while the Bistrian and Blackburn diet closely mirrors the keto diet. This is fascinating.

When a person is operating fully on glucose for energy, the level of oxygen intake is closely matched by the level of carbon dioxide (CO2) expelled. It is defined as a 1:1 ratio with metabolic testing.

If they are operating fully on fat for energy then the ratio is closer to 0.7. In other words for each litre of inhaled oxygen, 0.7 litres of CO2 is expelled. This is a more efficient process and has been explored by the US military as a benefit for deep sea diving.

This measurement called a Respiratory Quotient (RQ index), is able to be used, by a laboratory, to determine the actual proportions of fat and glucose being used for energy, because a person is always using a mix of these. It can identify when a person is unable to utilise body fat reserves and perhaps could help with diet planning. A healthy person should apparently be 80% fat burning while at rest.

Respiratory Quotient (RQ) Guide:

1.0   Diet mainly composed of Carbohydrates
0.8   Mixed Fat, Protein and Carbohydrates
0.7   Diet mainly composed of Fat.

Maria and Craig Emerich in their excellent book "Keto" reports a traditional living 25 year old Eskimo woman breast feeding after a 3-1/2 day fast who showed an RQ of 0.454. She was not only converting body fat for all her own energy including required glucose, she was also using her body fat to manufacture breast milk for the baby.

https://www.jbc.org/article/S0021-9258(18)83867-4/pdf

HOW DO WE GAIN BODY FAT?

With small meals and snacks all day, energy is coming in every few hours, or even more often, so your pancreas releases insulin regularly. When insulin levels are up, your body stores excess energy as fat and when insulin levels are very low, your body will release body fat for energy. Insulin is also known as the fat storage hormone. When you continually have high levels of insulin 'all day, every day', then your body responds by storing fat 'all day, every day'. Snacking drives the body to make insulin constantly and this drives up fat storage, locking out opportunities for release of your own stored fat.

Humans have a liking for food with a high fat and high carbohydrate combination, perhaps because it has such high energy levels. This type of food is very rare in nature, and existing only in human breast milk. Much of the processed food available today is low nutrition, processed food and is developed by food companies to exploit this liking and to encourage you to eat as much of it as possible. This is not surprising. Think about some examples: cakes, pizza, ice cream, donuts, cookies, cereals, bread with spreads, in fact almost all processed foods. This combination drives your body to eat more, resulting in any excess being stored as body fat. In addition, the oxidative priority, as described, will force your body to store fat when it has excess carbohydrate arriving. It is easy to overeat carbs for example being full after a main meal, but then you can still manage something sweet to finish.

A recommendation to eat any carbs near the end of the meal may assist with keeping your body processing fat for longer, before these rogue carbs arrive and screw up the whole process.

Not only are we programmed to like this carb and fat combination food, it is also incredibly cheap to produce because the main ingredients, sugar, corn and wheat are low cost and subsidised by the US government, making these processed foods incredibly profitable for the food companies. No wonder they are motivated to maintain the status quo and spend millions on advertising to encourage us to buy their products.

As well as this food being very attractive, the manufacturing process reduces protein and fibre so the resulting food is high in energy but low in nutrients. Sugar and wheat flour are perfect examples. The resulting low level of nutrients is believed to also drive over-eating as people unconsciously try to satisfy their protein appetite. When a farmer wants to fatten up an animal, they know to reduce the protein level of their feed and the animal will then eat more calories trying to get enough protein.

We expect to feel full when we've eaten sufficiently and no longer feel hunger pangs, but carbohydrates seem to bypass this feeling, with people being able to easily overeat on these. Fat and protein do not have this problem as they activate satiation sensors making you feel full prior to overeating. If you try eating lots of fat, you become sick of it very quickly.

With processed food that tastes amazing, snacking keeping insulin levels up continuously, low levels of protein plus carbs that fail to register your satiation sensors, the result is you can easily eat too much high energy food. The excess is stored as body fat, by the action of insulin, and this fat is seldom used.

There is yet another effect happening here. To contain this excess energy that has been stored as fat and prevent it from being released into the blood, your body must create higher and higher levels of insulin. If your body continually has high insulin levels it becomes adjusted to that particular level, and for the insulin hormone signalling to do its job, the level has to be raised even higher. Becoming adapted to a signal, is a common response by the body to many things, i.e. sunshine, bright light, bad smells, sweet tastes, drugs and loud noise, etc.

The requirement for higher levels of insulin is because of this 'insulin resistance' and it results in hyperinsulinemia, (continual high insulin levels) which is very harmful to your body. This condition causes blood vessel damage, macular degeneration in your eyes, obesity, nerve damage, brain damage, PCOS, and many problems that won't become evident for many years. It is termed 'metabolic syndrome' and, eventually, the continual high demand for insulin overloads the pancreas and leads to full type 2 diabetes. The recent availability of continuous glucose monitors (CGM) is now enabling people to see the real and immediate result of eating even moderate levels of sugars and starches.

A major failing of current medical testing for insulin resistance is that it focuses on the inability to get glucose into cells rather than checking how much insulin is being produced. The result being, that you could be sent away from the doctor after being told all is OK simply because the massive level of insulin in your body (hyperinsulinemia) manages glucose down, thereby, hiding the excess glucose problem. Unfortunately, the doctor may only realize there is a problem when the 'end-stage' symptoms start to show up some years later. Because excess insulin is causing serious micro-vascular damage during this undiagnosed period, much of the damage to your body may be irreversible by the end-stage.

If you have any concerns, you may be able to request full insulin resistance testing to avoid this problem. Thin people can also be severely insulin resistant, thin outside, fat inside (TOFI).

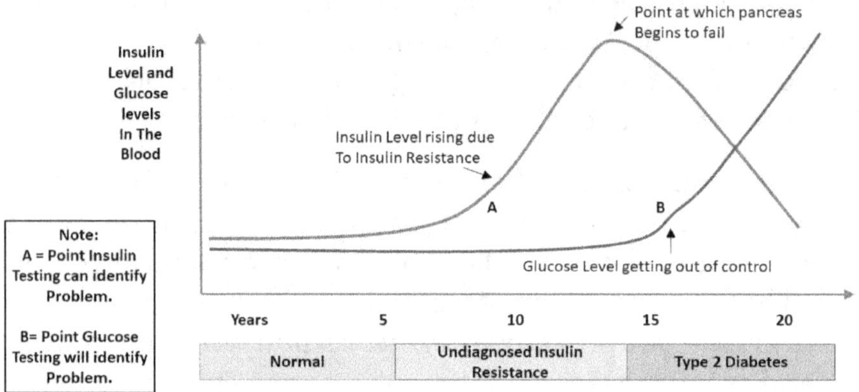

Too much insulin, too often, can have another very dangerous impact on the body.   Research has found that there is a clear link between higher insulin levels and the risk of cancer. For example, breast cancer cells have high numbers of insulin receptors. Research has shown that lowering insulin levels, can reduce your cancer risk.

One way your doctor could check on your insulin, is to request a C-Peptide test as C-Peptide is made by your body along with insulin but remains there for longer.   A normal range is 0.5 to 2.7 ng/mL. A very high level would indicate your pancreas is making lots of insulin but you may have insulin resistance, while a very low level might indicate Type-1 diabetes or Type-2 diabetes resulting from severe damage to the pancreas.

Here is a list of common insulin resistance symptoms:

- Increased body fat levels, particularly in the central area.

- Waist measurement greater than 35 inches for women and 40 inches for men. However, as mentioned you could be a TOFI, slim and still have severe insulin resistance.

- Increased levels of facial and body hair for women.

- Acanthosis Nigricans, a darkening of skin in folds, under arms and on backs of fingers. This can also be a serious indicator of cancer, diabetes, PCOS or other hidden problems.

- Difficulty getting pregnant, (applies to women only of course).

- Erectile disfunction, (applies to men only of course)

- Tendency to oily skin and hair, with an increased level of acne.

- Cravings for sweet or salty foods.

- Fatigue.

- Increased hunger or thirst.

- Skin tags, particularly around the neck and under arms which is a symptom of insulin promoting excess skin growth. Apparently some doctors are not sure what causes these.

I understand that when treating a Type 2 diabetes patient, some classically trained nutritionists or doctors will set a minimum level of carbohydrates that the patient must eat. Unfortunately for the patient, recent research has shown this to be an outdated approach as it continues to maintain unhealthy elevated insulin levels in their body with the associated damage that causes.

By advising a low carbohydrate diet instead, as was carried out historically, before the availability of synthetic insulin, and is undertaken today by many doctors including Dr. David Unwin in the UK, they may be able to put the disease into remission, as he is achieving with his patients. In 2016, he won the UK NHS National Innovator of the Year award for this pioneering work. In accepting the award, Dr David Unwin said:

> *"This great result helps show what a rewarding job general practice can be when we work together with our patients for better health. Diabetes is a national emergency, my patients have shown that many will choose healthy living over lifelong medication and that the low carb diet is one way to achieve that goal"*

Take a look here:

https://www.norwoodsurgerysouthport.nhs.uk/website/
N84008/files/
Press_release_low_Carb_GP_wins_National_Award.pdf

In New Zealand, Dr Glen Davies of Taupo, is treating Type-2 diabetes patients and pre-diabetic patients with a low carbohydrate diet. In 2020 he reported 100 patients in remission.

Check out:
https://lowcarbpractitioners.com/practitioner/davies/.

A great thing about treating metabolic syndrome with a low carbohydrate diet is how quickly results start to be seen. I have heard of patients reducing blood pressure medications significantly within days, reducing the fat level of a fatty liver by 30% in 1 week and improving overall metabolic measures within 3 weeks.

WHAT IS METABOLIC HEALTH?

This extract from the Low Carb High Fat dietitian (https://lchf-rd.com)

- Waist circumference: < 102 cm (40 inches) in men and 88 cm (34.5 inches) in women.
- Systolic Blood Pressure: < 120 mmHG
- Diastolic Blood Pressure: < 80 mmHG
- Glucose: < 5.5 mmol/L (< 100 mg/dL)
- HbA1c: < 5.7%
- Triglycerides: < 1.7 mmol/L (< 150 mg/dL)
- HDL cholesterol: >1.00 mmol/L (> 40 mg/dL) in men and > 1.30 mmol/L (> 50 mg/dL) in women.

Research from 2018 revealed that only 12% of American adults meet all these criteria and in Americans older than 60 years, only 2%. It is believed by some, that a major reason for the high death rate from COVID19 by older people was their poor metabolic health.

Stephen J. Guyenet Ph.D. in his book "The Hungry Brain" highlights from the 2010 USDA *Dietary Guidelines for Americans*, the top food calorie sources for US adults - in order:

1. Grain based desserts, (Donuts, cookies, cakes, etc)

2. Yeast breads

3. Chicken and chicken mix dishes (Fried chicken, nuggets, etc)

4. Soda / energy drinks/ sports drinks.

5. Alcoholic beverages

6. Pizza.

His list for children - in order is:

1. Grain based desserts

2. Pizza

3. Soda / energy drinks / sports drinks

4. Yeast breads

5. Chicken and chicken mix dishes

6. Pasta and pasta dishes.

Heavy sugar and high carbohydrate diets with low protein. Not ideal, and this list was compiled 10 years ago.

WHAT ABOUT SUGAR?

Sugar is a refined carbohydrate which triggers insulin production and the rise in insulin can be rapid. To remain healthy, it is necessary to minimize consumption of sugar particularly as it fails to trigger satiation sensors in your body. Carefully check nutrition labels on food to ensure minimal sugar, and look for the high number of substitute words manufacturers use to hide sugar. Sugar laden liquids such as soda's, soft drinks, fruit juice, and energy drinks are particularly dangerous because of their rapid absorption.

Fruit juice is perhaps the unhealthiest because it has very low fiber, lots of bad fructose (sugar), it is concentrated and very rapidly absorbed, massively spiking insulin levels in your body. That morning glass of orange juice at breakfast is a very unhealthy treat.

A glass of orange juice has a nutrient profile almost identical to a class of cola.

Many foods have been assigned a GI (Glycemic Index) value, which is designed to help us understand how quickly the food will spike insulin when digested. High GI foods that spike insulin rapidly include sugar, bread and products made from refined flour. Because fructose is metabolised differently in the body it does not spike insulin as quickly therefore has a lower GI score.

Carbohydrates are immediately converted to glucose (sugar) on digestion. Sugar can also create advanced glycation end products (AGE's) in our blood. This is where sticky sugar molecules stick to protein molecules in the blood and gum up the works, and the proteins are now said to be glycated. These can become too large to pass through the tiny blood vessels in the eyes and extremities. This problem is believed to contribute to blindness and gangrene infections in feet, toes and fingers of people with type 2 diabetes due to reduced blood flow to these areas. Fructose is 10x more effective than glucose at this. For more details see: https://pubs.acs.org/doi/pdf/10.1021/bi00406a016

Refined table sugar is approximately 50% sucrose and 50% fructose. Look out for High Fructose Corn Syrup (HFCS) on food labels, which comes in two forms with about 55% or 42% fructose. Manufacturers use many terms for sugar to hide it from you. Sometimes, the ingredients list on a processed food nutrition label will have multiple sugars listed, each one using a different name for sugar.

Sugar or fructose is often added to many processed foods when they are reformulated to be low-fat, in order to improve the taste.

In 2010 it was identified that fructose reacts differently to other sugars in the body becoming a potent stimulant for Non-Alcoholic Fatty Liver Disease, (NAFLD) which is thought to be a trigger for Metabolic Syndrome. Don't be fooled by the term 'fruit sugar', another name given to fructose, which is the most common sugar found in fruit. Your liver must immediately convert fructose into fat which puts a huge and immediate processing load on it.

The 'fructose' component of sugar is now believed, by some people, to be a poison in the body. If you are eating fruit, minimize quantities and make sure you eat the whole fruit and avoid fruit smoothies as they remove the fiber that helps slow digestion. Berries are a preferred fruit because of their lower levels of sugar, with strawberries and blueberries being amongst the best.

The recommended 'five plus per day' fruit and vegetables is a marketing ploy to encourage you to eat more fruit and vegetables and is not actually based on any solid science. Note that starchy foods like potatoes, convert directly to sugar in your body. A single 30-gram slice of white bread has the same insulin stimulation impact on the body as 3.7 teaspoons of sugar, while 150 grams of boiled potato has the same impact as 9.1 teaspoons of sugar. For those wishing to see what the sugar levels are in various foods, I recommend taking a look at Dr David Unwin's infographics at https://phcuk.org/sugar/

Of particular interest, is that cancer cells thrive on sugar and many cancers will not survive if there is no sugar available. Interestingly in laboratory experiments, cancer cells are fed glucose. To follow up take a look at this research https://www.ncbi.nlm.nih.gov/pmc/articles/PMC6375425/

Eating too many simple sugars is now known to increase the risk of developing depression with diabetics being 53% more likely to develop depression. In a study of 8,964 people, Spanish researchers sought to understand the relationship between eating sugary sweets and junk food and whether this could influence depression. Over a 6-year period, they determined that those who regularly consume junk food, were at a 37% greater risk of developing depression.

Should we be eating artificial sweeteners instead? Testing has shown that most of these still raise insulin levels and should be avoided. My advice to you is to train your taste buds to enjoy less sweet food.

I believe minimising sugar, especially fructose, is critical to maintaining your health. Paul McKenna in his book, 'Get control of sugar' calls sugar a slow-motion poison.

Food manufacturers can choose to replace sucrose with fructose in processed food in order to market a lower (Glycemic Index) GI product, but the result is actually worse for your health. Cancer cells can apparently learn to feed directly on fructose and proliferate.

Asians have been eating a high carbohydrate diet with rice for decades, but the recent massive in-crease in diabetes is thought to be directly attributable to the rise in their sugar consumption. In 1980 1% of Chinese had Type-2 diabetes, but one generation later, by 2013, 11.6% of Chinese adults have type 2 diabetes.

WHAT IS THE PROBLEM WITH WHEAT FLOUR?

Wheat has been a staple of some civilizations for many years. The Egyptians grew wheat alongside the Nile and ate flour as part of their standard diet. However, autopsies of mummies have revealed coronary artery disease and severe tooth decay.

The refining of wheat is similar to sugar refining, because the processing removes many of the nutrients resulting in low nutrition food but with higher calories. Furthermore, the presence of phytic acid (phytates) in wheat, react in the mouth causing tooth decay. It is perhaps not surprising to learn that based on the research of Weston A. Price, most traditional native groups had little if any tooth decay until they began to eat western type food.

Archeological records show that when humans changed from a hunter gatherer lifestyle to a predominately agricultural lifestyle, people became shorter with a reduced average lifespan of many years.

In the 1960's wheat was hybridized modifying it from the ancient varieties to modern varieties with larger seed heads and shorter strong stalks. In the process of this hybridization, they also changed the proteins and massively raised the level of gluten. It is believed that this change is what has driven the huge increase in coeliac disease and non-coeliac gluten sensitivity (NCGS).   Research suggests these two negative effects on the human body are believed to be responsible for a significant rise in human sickness.

One of the more insidious results of these negative effects is the damage done to the intestinal gut lining, increasing the risk of severe autoimmune diseases. These include arthritis, irritable bowel syndrome (IBS), Crohn's disease, leaky gut, many other gut diseases, and upwards of 120 different autoimmune diseases with very negative impacts on humans.

Many plants, plus wheat products and refined flour contain anti-nutrients. These are compounds that can attach to dietary nutrients and prevent their absorption by your body. For example: zinc, magnesium, iron and calcium can be impacted this way by the phytic acid found in wheat. There are also enzyme inhibitors in wholegrains that can stress the pancreas and other digestive processes causing allergies and digestive problems. Some animals that naturally feed on these products have complex multiple stomach digestive systems to ferment grains at an early stage of digestion. There are some traditional preparation approaches such as soaking, fermenting and sprouting that can minimise these problems, but most are not followed by modern diets. Sourdough bread is one exception to this.

Many cereals are manufactured by a high-pressure extrusion process that is suspected to seriously deplete much of the nutritional value. My research has unearthed some animal feeding studies that are generally ignored but suggest concerns with foods produced this way.

The bottom line is that most grain-based products including wheat are actually not particularly healthy for you. Eating processed flour in the many processed foods available today, immediately spikes a rush of glucose, triggering the release of insulin to manage it. 'Healthy wholegrains' are actually not healthy although they are slightly better than refined flour.

Any study of traditional people who have switched to western style diets of seed oils, sugar and flour reveals a massive reduction in general health, increased coronary heart disease, increased leaky gut and autoimmune diseases, tooth decay, type-2 diabetes, macular degeneration, obesity and cancers. Studies of Tokelau Islanders, Inuit and Australian Aborigines strongly suggest this.

LET'S LOOK AT FATS SOME MORE

Fats come in three main forms, saturated fat, monounsaturated fats and polyunsaturated fats as defined by their ability to bond to other elements. No food comes in a single fat form and all fats exist in combinations in the food that provides them.

For example:
- duck fat is 11% polyunsaturated, 56% monounsaturated and 27% saturated fat, whereas
- rice bran oil is 37% polyunsaturated, 38% mono saturated and 25% saturated fat.
- 100 grams of olive oil has 14 grams of saturated fat while 100 grams of steak has 8 grams.

Fats are identified by the availability of their molecular structures to link to other compounds. A saturated fat has no available links, a mono-unsaturated fat has 1 and a poly-unsaturated fat has 2 or more.

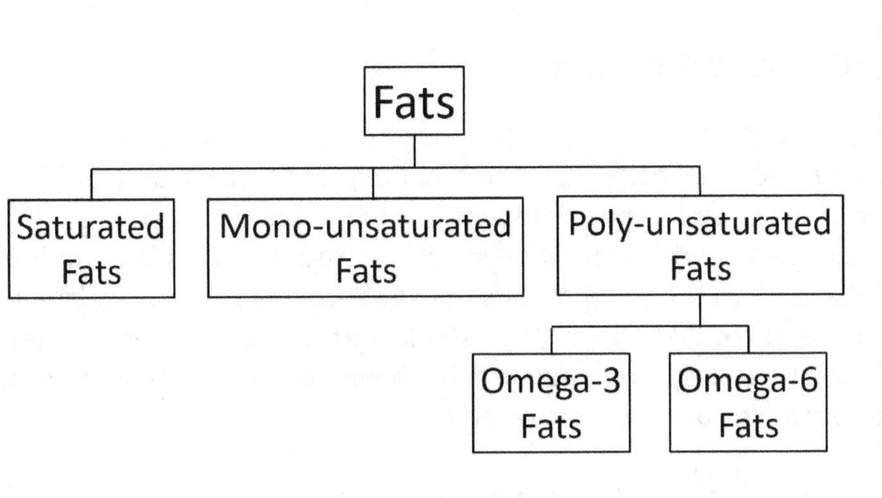

Fats
Saturated Fats
Mono-unsaturated Fats
Poly-unsaturated Fats
Omega-3 Fats
Omega-6 Fats

Saturated Fat (Sfa)

For about the last 50 years we have been advised to avoid saturated fats because it was believed that this fat could clog your arteries in the same way that fat sets when poured down a cold drain. It has now been discovered that this is completely false and, in fact, lower levels of saturated fat are unhealthy and can lead to a higher risk of strokes and many other problems. Unfortunately, some authorities have yet to assimilate this and continue to portray saturated fat as harmful.

50+ years of anti-fat sentiment has conditioned people to feel guilty, even fearful of eating it. Examples of foods with saturated fats include butter, olive oil, coconut oil, most cheeses and animal fats.

If you find this information hard to believe, then take a look at this article published in June 2020, by the American college of Cardiology, https://www.onlinejacc.org/content/early/2020/06/16/j.jacc.2020.05.077

Their summary: *Whole-fat dairy, unprocessed meat, and dark chocolate are SFA-rich foods with a complex matrix that are not associated with increased risk of CVD. The totality of available evidence does not support further limiting the intake of such foods.*

Gram for gram, olive oil has 14 times the total fat of beef and 2 times the level of saturated fat. Oily fish has 2 times the total fat and 1-1/2 times the saturated fat compared with red meat.

I read that in Gascony, France, the locals eat many duck dishes. Their diet is famously up to 35% saturated fat. The deaths from heart attacks is 50% that of the overall French level and 75% less than USA levels.

Here is the reworked conclusion of the 1966-73 Sydney Diet

Health Study, the results of which were initially suppressed, until recovered and made public 40 years later by CE Ramsden in 2013.

"Advice to substitute polyunsaturated fats for saturated fats is a key component of worldwide dietary guidelines for coronary heart disease risk reduction. However, clinical benefits of the most abundant polyunsaturated fatty acid, omega 6 linoleic acid, have not been established. In this cohort, substituting dietary linoleic acid (Omega-6 seed oils) *in place of saturated fats increased the rates of death from all causes, coronary heart disease, and cardiovascular disease. An updated meta-analysis of linoleic acid* (Industrial seed oils) *intervention trials, showed no evidence of cardiovascular benefit. These findings could have important implications for worldwide dietary advice to substitute omega 6 linoleic acid, or polyunsaturated fats in general, for saturated fats."*

So, for 40 years the results of an important study on the effects, of replacing saturated fats with polyunsaturated industrial seed oils (vegetable oils), were known to be much less healthy for people and, this information was suppressed.

Monounsaturated Fat (Mufa)

These fats are generally considered healthy and are a major component of olive oil which is a part of a recommended 'Mediterranean diet'. They are seen as 'good' fats. Just be careful when buying these to ensure they are pure without dilution from unhealthy oils.

Pure Olive oil is 73% Monounsaturated fat. This fat is known as Oleic acid and is found in olive oil and in Bacon.

Analysis of some low-cost olive oils in USA, has found more than half of them to be contaminated with canola oil. It has become common, particularly in Europe for olive oils to be diluted with lower cost vegetable oils often while still advertising them as extra-virgin. This trend is reducing the quality of olive oils because the added vegetable oils are polyunsaturated, which increases the level of oxidation and promotes inflammation within the body. These lower cost oils are forcing down overall quality as ethical suppliers find that unless they also dilute, their pure oils are priced out of the market.

While there are defined standards for these oils, it seems that they are mostly ignored with only Australian authorities regularly inspecting local products to ensure compliance.

Polyunsaturated Fat (Pufa)

These fats come predominantly in 2 forms, Omega-3 (alpha-linolenic acid) and Omega-6 (linoleic acid). Both of these are necessary for your health, but only in tiny quantities and they must be balanced. Omega-3 reduces inflammation while Omega-6 stimulates inflammation in your body. Unfortunately, in the early 1900's manufacturers found they could extract Omega-6 oils from seeds by crushing, soaking in chemicals (hexane), bleaching deodorizing etc. and bottling these seed oils to sell.   They are cheap and advertised as healthy, (labelled as vegetable oils to make them sound good) but subsequent testing has shown that they can be very toxic to humans.

One of the earliest of these products was marketed and sold as 'Crisco' a purported healthier replacement for the common animal sourced fats, Butter, lard, tallow, and suet used in home cooking at that time. These days they are sold as the many different liquid cooking (vegetable) oils and margarine.

Many trials have found serious health issues resulting from consumption of these including increased cancers in test subjects, believed to be linked to increased inflammation from Omega-6 seed oil consumption. Because Polyunsaturated oils have multiple double bonds in the molecular structure, they readily oxidise (go rancid) to create toxic compounds.

Dr. Wolfgang Lutz, an Austrian physician born in 1913 and an early diet researcher, found that these seed oils were not well tolerated by Crohn's sufferers.

It took 20 years from Ignaz Semmelweis first demonstration of the benefits of hand washing until it became standard practise before surgery and I fear it will take even longer to accept the dangers of excess of Omega-6 oils. To date the only form of these oils restricted is trans-fats, which are hydrogenated or partially hydrogenated Omega-6 oils. However, while trans-fats are recognised as dangerous, the US FDA allows manufacturers to label their products as having zero trans fats if the level is less than 0.5 grams per serving. How many servings are in a packet of cookies?

A prominent nutrition researcher, Dr Paul Mason of Australia, states that eating excess Omega-6 seed oils is equivalent to smoking 2 packs of cigarettes per day. However, it is very difficult to avoid these inflammatory industrial seed oils which include: corn oil, soya bean oil, rape seed oil, grape seed oil, cotton seed oil, sunflower oil, safflower oil, canola oil, in fact any oils made from seeds, as they are an ingredient of many processed foods. Take a look at the ingredients in any processed food nutrition panel. They are often called vegetable oils, but this is just a marketing term as they are all manufactured from seeds. I suggest you avoid them, as some testing has shown that they can severely increase your risk of cancer.

When you eat a serving of fries cooked in vegetable oils, you are getting a huge carbohydrate load (potato) coated in toxic oils, a recipe for a massive increase in body fat storage and inflammation in your body. Because the toxicity of these oils increases as they are repeatedly heated and cooled, the oil used in restaurant fryers can be especially toxic. If you want to know why I am so concerned about the risk with seed oils, take a look at: https://Youtu.be/7kGnfXXIKZM

Omega-3 (PUFA) oils can also go rancid easily. These mostly come from egg yolks, fish, and a little from flax seed, but importantly, can help reduce inflammation in your body. Minimizing Omega-6 oils and getting as much Omega-3 as possible is desirable. Traditional diets would typically have a ratio of about 1:1 of these 2 oils, whereas modern diets now have huge excesses of Omega-6 oils because they are in most processed food and used by most restaurants and homes to fry food.

It is reported that for some teenagers their ratio of Omega-6 PUFA to Omega-3 PUFA is as high as 40 : 1.

In 2015, testing of a range of fish-oil supplements in New Zealand found most were already rancid (oxidised). I would not recommend using these supplements to increase Omega-3 intake, instead eat whole small fatty fish such as sardines.

https://pubmed.ncbi.nlm.nih.gov/25604397/

One reason for the huge use of this toxic oil is the incorrect fear of saturated fat. Once we get past this huge error in understanding, food may revert to saturated fat and general health should improve. There is speculation that the rise in PUFA fat under the skin is behind the huge rise in skin cancers which closely matches the rise in PUFA consumption.

Polyunsaturated seed oils (vegetable oils or PUFA's) have gone from only 1% of the USA Diet in 1900 to 80grams, or 32% of the caloric intake in 2010.

IS BACON OK?

Should we be concerned about nitrites or nitrates in bacon? Meat retailers are experiencing a downturn in demand for bacon due to resistance from people who are concerned about health risks of eating meat. Let's examine this.

The plant-based lobby is working hard to discredit animal-based foods despite our ancestors regularly eating meat or fish, often as the only food consumed. The dominance of these animal and fish based diets over thousands of years have been confirmed by isotope testing of human remains (Richard's M.P. et al. 2009) and are still the basis of a number of traditional diets for groups such as the Masai, Inuit, Hadza and Tokelau Islanders.

These groups, eating traditional diets, do not apparently suffer from the cancers common amongst people eating a modern diet. It is revealing to note that as these people migrate to a more western diet, their health declines. The Australian aborigines and Pima Indians of Arizona are well documented examples of this change from predominantly meat based diets to western diets and their resulting health issues.

In 1906-12, American doctor and anthropologist, Vilhjalmur Stefansson, lived with the Inuit in Northern Canada for about 5 years eating their nearly 100% animal based diet of fish, caribou, whale, seal and other smaller animals without any significant health issues. He recorded their good health and longevity and noted in his diaries and books that he very rarely observed any cancer.

Dietary comparison is difficult due to the number of confounding factors. For example, vegetarians and vegans are often very particular about what they eat meaning that a study finding benefits from their diet may be unable to establish if the benefit came from eating vegetables or from avoiding sugar, alcohol, processed foods or refined grains. In addition, meat eaters as a group often include people who are less concerned about their diet, seldom exercise, consume alcohol frequently and eat lots of processed food, all of which can contribute to poor health. Is a diet with plenty of hamburgers bad because of the meat or the bun?

Colon cancer is sometimes linked to meat consumption and there are studies about this. However, a UK study (Tim Key, 2022) examined data on 63,550 men and women aged 20 to 89 recruited throughout the UK during the 1990s. They obtained the cancer incidence figures from national cancer registries. They concluded: *"Within the study, the incidence of all cancers combined was lower (11%) among vegetarians than among meat eaters, but the incidence of colorectal cancer was higher in vegetarians (39%) than in meat eaters."*

One of the concerns raised about eating bacon is the presence of Nitrates and Nitrites initially present in the meat and added for the curing process, to preserve the meat, extend the shelf life, and to keep it looking red and delicious. They suppress the bacteria that causes Botulism in meat and, without them, the meat can look grey and unappealing.

Nitrates (NO_3) are relatively stable and, therefore, in small quantities they are unlikely to change and cause harm, however bacteria and enzymes in the mouth will convert them to nitrites.

The nitrites are then converted by stomach acid to Nitric Oxide (NO). This is beneficial.

Nitrites (NO2) which come into contact with protein are converted to nitric oxide which is very beneficial for the body and is a natural anti-bacterial. This helps lower blood pressure, helps people with angina, and relaxes artery walls, assisting with blood circulation and is the active compound in Viagra. Nitrites are not stable and in the 1970's it was suggested that heating them can create Nitrosamines which can be carcinogenic. The good news is that these nitrosamines are heat-labile, ie: altered or destroyed by high heat (Am J Clin Nutr. - 2009).

Curiously people are less concerned about nitrates and nitrites in vegetables, which is where 80% of the ingested nitrates and nitrites come from, according to the above study. Beetroot greens and juice are touted as health foods because of the abundant nitrites which convert into Nitric Oxide when eaten. Celery for example, is very high in nitrites, can be ground into a powder and used as a replacement preservative in processed meats. When this is done the meat, must by (US) law, be labelled as "uncured".

There is no difference in the action of the nitrites regardless of the source. The craziness is that (in USA) when the nitrite comes from sodium (or potassium) nitrite, it's regulated (allowable levels vary by product). There are no limits for nitrite from celery powder, which means that bacon labelled as "uncured" may actually contain higher levels of nitrites. It turns out that almost all meat labelled "uncured" has been treated with vegetable based nitrites.

Nitrites are also present in drinking water and naturally occur in saliva, where they function as an anti-bacterial with, for example, the ability to kill salmonella. Nitrite in saliva increases gastric mucosal blood flow and mucus thickness helping digestion. This action removes toxins, and helps with acid buffering by supporting bicarbonate production downstream of the stomach.

The summary of one study claimed: *"These results indicate that dietary nitrate may serve important gastro-protective functions".*

In a study (N P Sen, et al. 1980) the nitrosamine levels detected in both cured and uncured meat products (both cooked and uncooked) were very low and were degraded and destroyed by cooking at high heat and, therefore, would not be expected to occur in fried foods at significant levels.

Like most dietary substances there are upper limits. Excess nitrate (NO3) which has no taste or smell, can affect how our blood carries oxygen. Nitrates can turn hemoglobin (the protein in blood that carries oxygen) into methemoglobin . High levels can turn skin to a bluish or gray-color and cause more serious health effects like weakness, excess heart rate, fatigue, and dizziness. This is sometimes referred to as "blue baby syndrome" as babies are particularly vulnerable. In some US farm areas warnings are issued when nitrate levels get too high in drinking water.

In New Zealand, if nitrate (NO3) levels in drinking water exceed 50 mg/L, then it must be treated. Boiling or disinfectant has zero impact on this. Generally, only private bore water would have this problem with rain water unlikely to be affected and community supply water regularly tested for this.

One study (Dubrow et al. 2010) examined 545,000 participants of which 585 were diagnosed with Glioma, (Brain Tumours). They were testing the hypothesis that Nitrosamines derived from dietary Nitrites (NO2) elevated the risk of brain tumours. Their conclusions stated:

"We found no significant trends in glioma risk for consumption of processed or red meat, nitrate, or vitamin C or E. We found significant positive (not good) *trends for nitrite intake from plant sources and, unexpectedly, for fruit and vegetable intake. Further work is needed on early life diet, adult intake of nitrite from plant sources, and adult intake of fruit and vegetables in relation to adult glioma risk".* *"We observed an unexpected finding of increasing glioma risk with increasing intake of fruit and vegetables. ~~~ which may be due to pesticide residues consumed with fruit and vegetables"*

What about the fat in bacon? The fats in bacon are about 50% monounsaturated and a large part of those is oleic acid. This is the same fatty acid present in olive oil and is generally considered "heart-healthy". The remaining fat in bacon is 40% saturated and 10% polyunsaturated, accompanied by some cholesterol. Dietary cholesterol was a concern in the past, but scientists now agree that it has very minor effects on cholesterol levels in your blood, while the Sydney Diet Health study showed us that saturated fat is healthy.

Maybe bacon does not need to be avoided?

CHOLESTEROL

In the late 60's, there was an outcry about the number of deaths from Coronary Vascular Disease (CVD) which had increased significantly over the previous decades. A study of heart attack victims showed a high level of cholesterol at the damage sites which led to the conclusion that the high cholesterol was causing the problem. As a result, guidelines were introduced to limit cholesterol and doctors began testing cholesterol levels in patients. Drug companies began to design cholesterol lowering drugs and cholesterol levels were considered the major indicator of heart attack risk.

There is no such thing as LDL cholesterol or HDL cholesterol, cholesterol is just cholesterol. Cholesterol is a fat, and must be packaged within a complex particle called a lipoprotein, in order to enable it to be transported within blood, which is water based.

There are a range of lipoproteins, from large to small, known as Very Low-Density Lipoprotein (VLDL), Intermediate-Density Lipoprotein (IDL), Low-Density Lipoprotein (LDL) and High-Density Lipoprotein (HDL). All of these lipoproteins can transport cholesterol as can red blood cells (RBC). When someone says LDL cholesterol (or LDL-C) they are actually referring to an LDL particle carrying cholesterol.

Cholesterol is critical for many functions in the body including operation of your immune system, your nerves and your brain plus the synthesis of hormones. Without it you will die.

Your liver makes the Very Low-Density Lipoproteins (VLDL) as a way of ferrying fatty-acids and cholesterol, via your blood, to different cells in the body. These fats must be transported in lipoproteins in blood, as blood is water based and wont mix with fats. The VLDL particles are loaded with Triglycerides, Cholesterol and other compounds for distribution.

The major source of the fatty-acids is excess dietary carbohydrates, proteins and alcohol that have been converted into fatty-acids by a process called De novo lipogenesis. The liver is actively trying to get rid of these fatty-acids. As the VLDL carrier deposits fatty-acids and cholesterol at each site around the body, it shrinks eventually becoming the size referred to as a Low-Density Lipoprotein (LDL). When it has delivered its load of fatty-acids and cholesterol, it returns to the liver and the process begins again.

Accordingly, when you eat excess carbohydrate your LDL level will rise and a low carbohydrate diet means your LDL level will usually fall. The (HDL) High Density Lipoprotein carries unused cholesterol from body tissues back to the liver. The impact of saturated fats on cholesterol levels is more fully explained further on in the book.

The surface of the LDL lipoprotein has a single copy of a receptor protein known as Apo B-100 which is like a key identifying the lipoprotein to each location as required, including to the liver on its return. If this receptor should become damaged in any way, then the particle is not recognized by any of the locations and it becomes an orphan particle.

There are a number of ways this receptor can be damaged with glycation being one and oxidation another. Excess sugar in the blood can drive glycation and oxidative stress and oxidized oils in the diet, can drive oxidation of the LDL particle and receptor.

There are different theories about how atherosclerosis forms on artery walls, with the dominant theory called 'The Diet-Heart Cholesterol Hypothesis'. In brief, this theory posits that saturated fat raises LDL cholesterol levels, which can become oxidized and can then penetrate artery walls causing damage. The body attempts to repair this damage resulting in arterial plaques.

These plaques can build up eventually closing off arteries and, if they detach from the artery walls, can cause blockages in critical parts of the body, such as the heart or brain. Depriving arteries of a blood supply can result in cell death followed by heart attack or stroke.

In a variation on this view, Professor Vladimir Subbotin has suggested that oxidized LDL cholesterol gets into your artery wall, not from inside the artery through the endothelial layer as usually proposed but, by being deposited there from the outside by the blood that supplies the artery walls. His argument is very compelling and, if true, indicates a sequence whereby an offending factor causes the initial thickening of arterial walls in the intima, which lies just behind the blood facing endothelial layer. This thickness calls for an additional blood supply which is provided by blood vessels feeding the artery walls (vasa vasorum) and growing into the intima layer. Oxidized LDL particles can accumulate at that point. Professor Subbotin posits that the commonly presented endothelial layer, as a single cell layer, is flawed, instead growing from birth into a 25-30 cell layer by about the age of 30.

A key driver for his view is that early stage oxidized LDL particle deposits occur at the endothelial / media junction multiple layers down from the glycocalyx rather than behind the surface endothelial layer. At these sites the blood vessels have already grown to supply the area with blood.

The glycocalyx is a fine hairlike layer on the inside surface of the blood vessels, only about 20 nanometers thick, that make them slippery, very much like the slippery layer on fish skin.

The Diet-Heart Cholesterol theory posits that the artery walls can become 'sticky' by the action of contaminants in the blood, such as excess sugars, glycation or oxidized PUFA causing inflammation. This stickiness damages the glycocalyx and encourages oxidized LDL particles to adhere to the walls, starting the process of atherosclerosis. The damage in the artery walls then forms plaque. These plaques are the beginning of atherosclerosis eventually leading to arterial blockages and Cardio Vascular Disease (CVD).

Findings now suggest that higher levels of LDL can assist in regression of these plaques, whereas lower levels of LDL assist plaque progression. This matches the concept of cholesterol as part of both the immune system and the repair process.

Where does the oxidation come from? The most prevalent source of oxidization is believed to be oxidized Omega-6 seed oils (PUFA). It is nearly impossible for seed oils not to be oxidized and, greater oxidative stress in the body has been consistently measured following vegetable oil consumption in the diet. In contrast, saturated fats have a molecular structure that renders them very stable and unlikely to become oxidized, which means that they do not contribute to oxidative stress.

A suggested measure of oxidative stress is the ratio of HDL to triglycerides in your blood, using US units (mg/dL). Triglyceride level divided by HDL level will produce a result which ideally should be under 1.5 or better still close to 1.0.

Using my personal blood test result as an example,
Triglycerides = 62 mg/dL (0.7 mmol/L/)
HDL = 74 mg/dL (1.92 mol/L)
Ratio Trig / HDL = 62 / 74 = 0.84 (= good)

Apparently, research has identified that the Vegan diet will reduce HDL and raise Triglycerides which indicates an increase in oxidative stress from this diet. While researchers often cite the reduction in LDL that this diet causes as a good result, it is believed by other researchers that while the overall LDL has decreased, the level of oxidized LDL has significantly increased.

In an adjustment to the Diet-Heart Cholesterol Hypothesis, it is now considered that only cholesterol in oxidized LDL, sometimes referred to as small dense LDL, progresses the formation of plaques in arteries and this is primarily driven by inflammation, and oxidation, while non-oxidized LDL cholesterol (referred to as large fluffy LDL), is not a driver of atherosclerosis and may not deserve its label as bad cholesterol.

Inexplicably, low cholesterol levels are correlated with higher rates of overall mortality (not lower). In people over 60, higher cholesterol is in fact, more healthy, particularly in women. This is the opposite of conventional understanding. UK Dr. Zoe Harcombe PhD. has produced some great graphics by gender, showing deaths per 100,000 people vs cholesterol levels using WHO data from 192 countries, which clearly show this correlation.

Dr. Zoe Harcombe PhD. also states "*Ancel Keys, the same man who did the brilliant Minnesota starvation experiment, spent the 1950's trying to show that cholesterol in food was associated with cholesterol in the blood. He concluded unequivocally that there was not even an association, let alone a causation. He never deviated from this view.*"

Cholesterol is a critical part of your immune system and this helps explain why LDL levels drop when people get infections. Cholesterol is an antioxidant, which could be the reason it rises as we age. Cholesterol at Cardio Vascular Disease (CVD) sites is now believed by many to help repair the artery damage and is not the cause of the problem.

There is an alternative view as to the cause of Atherosclerosis, and this view, called the Thrombogenic Process, seems to better fit the available evidence however, it has been actively suppressed, possibly because it doesn't support the hugely profitable market for cholesterol lowering medications and low-fat foods. This view is well described with excellent references by Dr. Malcolm Kendrick in his book "The Clot Thickens".

The Thrombogenic Process posits that various actions can damage the artery walls such as pollutants in the blood, high blood pressure, sickle cells, and other conditions that damage the glycocalyx (the slippery hairlike lining of the artery walls). These insults can arise from inflammation, high blood sugar, smoking, raised blood pressure, insulin resistance, steroid use, rheumatoid arthritis, toxins and many other causes. This damage produces blood clots (Thrombus) which can be as small as a rice grain, which then become plaques as the body sets about repairing the damage.

Blood clots draw in platelets and red blood cells that are rich in cholesterol and fibrin which build up the plaques. As part of the coagulation cascade, endothelial progenitor cells are attracted to the damage and build a new endothelium (artery wall layer) over the blood clot.

Finally, the presence or absence of Nitric oxide (NO) is important because it relaxes the artery, dilates blood vessels, prevents particles sticking to the glycocalyx and is a powerful anti-coagulant. It is also essential for erectile function suggesting that ED is a serious warning of impending atherosclerosis. NO is manufactured in the skin during exposure to sunlight. Low NO levels which are prevalent in people with insulin resistance will, therefore, exacerbate the risk of blood clots (thrombus). This also suggests that any condition that makes your blood less likely to clot is protective. High NO levels and daily aspirin fit this concept.

The problems resulting from blocked arteries or detached

plaques can then cause heart attacks or strokes in line with other theories.

Cholesterol is not the villain in this theory, however, all the mechanisms that may cause artery wall (endothelium layer) damage do come into play.

It then follows that if you have a healthy glycocalyx, you have a major protective barrier against endothelial damage, formation of blood clots and cardiovascular disease.

How then does Type-2 diabetes lead to heart disease? By reducing nitric oxide synthesis, increasing endothelial damage, increasing blood coagulation, reducing the level of endothelial progenitor cells, damaging the glycocalyx and increasing glycation damage throughout the body.

Maybe it is time to update our understanding of heart disease. The glycocalyx was only identified in 1963 and seen for the first time with an electron microscope in 1966. The ability of the endothelial cells to make NO was not understood until 1986, although it was recognized in 1980 that something was being produced that was relaxing blood vessel walls. Endothelial progenitor cells in the blood were not identified until 1997. Up until then, it was assumed that existing endothelial cells spread from the edges of a plaque.

Based on these various scenarios and the many hours of reading and review, I now lean strongly towards the Thrombogenic Process. There are some important clues as to its accuracy. Just as water comes in different forms of ice, steam and liquid, cholesterol also comes in different forms. Apparently the dominant form of cholesterol found in atherosclerotic plaques is not the form found in LDL particles, but it can be derived from the cholesterol found in red blood cells. The rapid action, by the eEndothelial progenitor cells, to build new endothelium over the plaque creates the appearance that the cholesterol has arrived from the vasa vasorum which aligns with the theory from Professor Vladimir Subbotin.

I believe that the strong efforts being taken to cancel Dr. Malcolm Kendrick, signal his message is no doubt true and a real threat to the massive drug profits from cholesterol lowering drugs. There are far too many inconsistencies with The Diet-Heart Cholesterol Hypothesis, such as the longer life span of women with higher cholesterol, the lack of any sort of progress reducing CVD following decades of cholesterol lowering medication, and large surveys (https:// pubmed.ncbi.nlm.nih.gov/19081406/) finding that at least half the people admitted to hospital with CVD have average or low cholesterol levels. Strangely, instead of concluding that high cholesterol may not actually drive up CVD risk, they choose to double down on the diet-heart cholesterol theory suggesting the need for further reductions in cholesterol levels!

We have already discovered that cholesterol in our food has almost zero impact on the level in the body which explains why early recommendations to limit egg consumption have been dropped. We also understand that the saturated fat (SAT) we eat, has no link to LDL particles as it comes into the blood directly from the intestinal tract, packed in chylomicrons, not LDL. We know that plant sterols in omega-6 polyunsaturated seed oils (vegetable oils) can displace cholesterol in human membranes and that people with high levels of plant sterols can suffer from sitosterolemia which usually causes advanced severe atherosclerosis.

People replacing excess omega-6 polyunsaturated fats with saturated fats will reduce the plant sterols and, as a consequence, increase their cholesterol level. I believe that this is a good thing as it is returning the body to how it is supposed to be and just like temperature, oxygen saturation, hydration and salt levels, cholesterol is probably being managed by the body to an optimum level for you.

People are starting to resist prescribed cholesterol lowering drugs, such as statins, due to side effects and some recent evidence showing little benefit. Prescription of these drugs might be because of standard practice 'rules' that require this, rather than because it is actually beneficial for your health.

So if cholesterol is not a risk factor, what should you be looking for? My research suggests that the best indicator is your Triglycerides level which is elevated if you have a higher risk of coronary artery disease but low if you do not. The target level is less than 1.70 mmol/L (USA units, below 150 mg/dl).

Below is a graph showing how large fluffy (Good LDL) cholesterol reduces as the triglyceride levels increase and then the small dense (Bad, Oxidised) cholesterol levels rise.

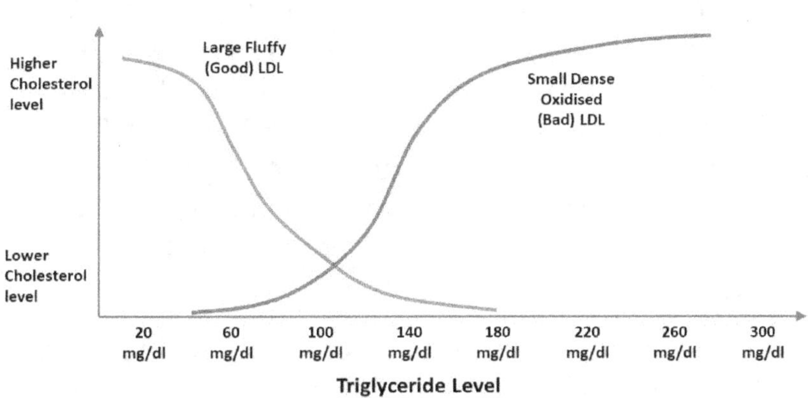

Plants also have a form of cholesterol used in the cellular membranes, which are collectively known as Phytosterols, sometimes referred to as 'plant sterols'. It has been noted that increased consumption of plant sterols can lead to lowered levels of cholesterol and the mechanism for this is believed to be that it inhibits intestinal absorption of cholesterol. As a result, it has been seen as positive, to increase this in diets that are seeking to reduce cholesterol. Plant sterols are present in all plants, but particularly concentrated in seed oils with the highest concentrations in rice bran oil (1891mg/100g), rape seed oil (canola) (893) and corn oil (990). Lower levels exist in olive oil (288mg/100g), Soy oil (355) and walnut oil (272).

The resulting drop in blood cholesterol may be due to the phytosterol simply replacing cholesterol, which may be even less healthy.

This mechanism can explain why increasing your consumption of saturated fat can raise cholesterol. The diet change is replacing "plant sterols" from polyunsaturated fats with real cholesterol, arguably a good change.

Some research has found that high amounts of plant sterols, while reducing overall cholesterol levels, correlates with increased risk of strokes and heart disease. One of the negative impacts of replacing cholesterol with phytosterols is observed in red blood cells (RBC) where a standard cell can easily deform to fit through microscopic blood vessels such as in eyes and extremities. In comparison, an RBC with a high level of phytosterols becomes more rigid, resisting the deformation required to pass through microscopic blood vessels, creating blockages and reducing the required level of blood nourishment to the tissues.

This doubt about the health benefits of increased phytosterols has resulted in the UK, France and Germany now discouraging advice to use phytosterols for heart disease prevention.

A side note:

"Phyto..." is a prefix used to indicate that a substance is sourced from plants. As a result plants provide phyto-nutrients while animal based foods do not. However this is just a naming trick, the same nutrients are often even more available from animal foods with greater bio-availability, but they are just not given the name Phyto.......

DAIRY

Dairy can be a good source of protein and has a high level of saturated fat (SFA). But we now know that dietary saturated fat is actually good for us. A recent report claimed a higher consumption of dietary SFA is associated with a lower risk of stroke, and every 10 g/day increase in SFA intake is associated with a 6% relative risk reduction in the rate of stroke. https://doi.org/10.1016/j.numecd.2019.09.028

Liquid milk contains milk sugar (lactose) which is a sugar (carbohydrate) and therefore if you want to avoid carbs for the reasons outlined previously, then avoid liquid milk. Solid milk such as cheese, butter and heavy cream, does not contain this lactose so is all perfectly okay on a low carb diet, plus you are getting good fats. It is quite a mind shift to think that cream might be more healthy than milk.

Some people cannot tolerate milk and react to the A1 protein, known as beta-casein, and they should avoid milk. This is often called 'lactose intolerance' and is more pronounced in non-European sourced populations that don't have the historical exposure to this A1 protein. However, there are cow breeds that produce only A2 protein instead and there is a program by some milk companies to breed more A2 cows, increasing the amount of A2 protein milk available. Goats milk only contains the A2 protein.

Some people have a view that cows milk is only a food for young cows and, therefore, is not an appropriate food for people. Humans are the only mammal that drinks the milk of another mammal. Some believe that raw milk is healthier than pasteurised, but I worry that if the collection process is not perfectly clean then we may be ingesting pathogens in the milk.

Only about 1/3 of the calcium in cows milk is absorbable by a human, the remainder is filtered out by your kidneys. If you are drinking milk for bone health, then you can do much better with leafy greens or certain types of fish. Read the chapter: Is Grass Finished Better? Osteoporosis is higher in women from countries that have high milk consumption. Those with the strongest bones often don't drink milk at all and surprisingly, hip fracture rates seem to be highest in countries drinking the most milk. Milk also has a negative impact on prostate cancer in men, more milk equates to more prostate cancer.

For an understanding of why the lysine in dairy is beneficial, see the chapter titled "Fighting a Virus".

SALT AND SUPPLEMENTS

Just like we got cholesterol wrong, we seem to have been wrong about salt. Examination of the basis for the original dietary salt restrictions reveals serious flaws in the research. Recent research has identified that low salt levels increase health risk much more than high salt levels. A new study of thousands of people around the world has identified that there is an optimum level of salt consumption (3-6 grams sodium per day) which is higher than current recommended levels.

The Japanese diet is very high in salt and they have one of the longest life expectancies in the world. We need salt for many internal body processes including digestion, manufacture of bile, hormone production, it is critical for brain function and may be a mood booster.

We now have to be aware of micro-plastics in salt made from evaporated sea water with 90% of salt produced this way showing some contamination, particularly high in Asia. A salt substitute from "Senomyx" is entering the food chain without any testing and can be called "artificial flavour" on food labels.

To follow the research check here: https://www.nejm.org/doi/

full/10.1056/NEJMoa1311889

The concern linking excess salt to raised blood pressure is apparently over stated with higher salt making a very small difference to blood pressure levels. My research suggests that lower salt may assist about 30% of people by dropping blood pressure a very small amount (1-4 mmHg), but for 20%, blood pressure will rise while for the remainder, there will be no change at all. High sugar levels in the blood, are now believed to drive up blood pressure.

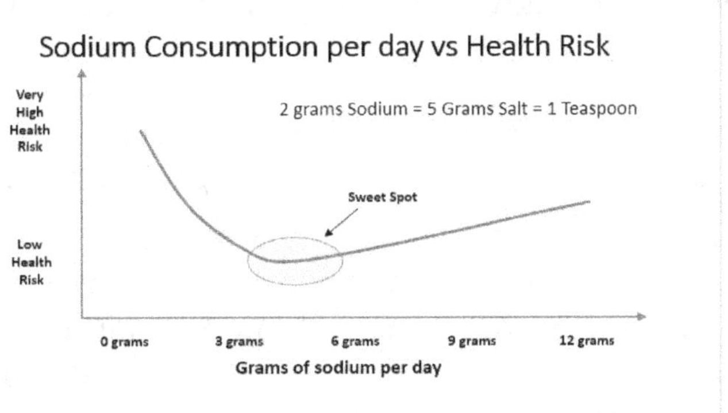

On a Keto or low carbohydrate diet, the reduction in insulin causes the kidneys to release more salt in urine and this coupled with the lower salt intake from the reduction in the consumption of processed food, usually reduces dietary salt levels. For some people this connection between lower insulin levels and reduced salt retention can help reduce blood pressure. Surprisingly, this is not well understood, despite being known since 1970's.

If sodium is low, your body will excrete potassium to keep these in sync which can be dangerous. For some people this salt loss can cause them to suffer from mild leg cramps and they may need to supplement salt to control this.

For women particularly, studies have shown that low salt levels can reduce bone health, increasing osteoporosis and the risk of hip fracture. https://pubmed.ncbi.nlm.nih.gov/30228731/.

You can expect to supplement salt on a keto or low carbohydrate diet and most days I add 1/2 tsp salt to a morning glass of water to keep levels up.

A study of the impact of salt levels in people with pre-diabetes (type-2) found that low salt reduced insulin sensitivity meaning that a low-salt diet can condition the body to need an even higher level of insulin in order to control glucose levels. (https://DOI: 10.1210/jcem.83.5.4835). This is alarming because common advice to minimize salt may be increasing diabetes risk.

Taking a look at other supplements.

Meat contains all the essential amino acids (Proteins) necessary for life, all the essential fats, and twelve of the thirteen essential vitamins in surprisingly large quantities. Meat is a particularly concentrated source of vitamins A and E, and the entire complex of B vitamins. Vitamins B12 and D are found only in animal products (although we may get vitamin D from regular exposure to sunlight).

James E. Dowd M.D. in his book, "The Vitamin D cure" (2008), highlights that the majority of people in USA, are deficient in vitamin D which he believes contributes to many health problems. He has case studies in which changing diets including reduction of refined grains and supplementing with vitamin D has provided huge benefits to his patients. He is particularly concerned to ensure that unborn babies and young children get sufficient vitamin D to set them up for a healthy adult life.

We are seeing a resurgence of interest in this with the concern that lack of Vitamin D contributes to worse outcomes for COVID-19. Recommendations from some sources are now suggesting up to 4000 iu per day.

Care must be taken with calcium supplements. Researchers have identified that when calcium is supplemented without vitamin D, the result can be an increase in the risk of cardiovascular disease due to calcium build up in arteries. A better approach may be to take vitamin K2 instead which has been proven to reduce bone loss due to ageing and also assist in the removal of calcium from soft tissue. See https://www.ncbi.nlm.nih.gov/pmc/articles/PMC4566462/

B vitamins supplementation is often required, particularly by vegans, and non-fortified nutritional yeast is one recommended source. Apparently, this is not always recognized by GP's, with some people suffering from low Vitamin B levels, taking years to have the problem identified.

Fat soluble vitamins A, D, E and K can only be absorbed by the body if there is fat available in the diet, without this, the vitamins will just pass through the body. Supplements with these vitamins often state that they must be taken with food. The B vitamins and vitamin C are water soluble but any excess is unable to be stored by the body so must be included in the diet regularly.

It has been discovered recently that vitamin C needs are much lower in people who are 'fat-burners', perhaps because there is vitamin C in meat fat. This may explain why people eating fresh meat with full fat have a low to zero requirement for vitamin C supplements to avoid scurvy. The traditional Inuit diet of nearly 100% meat and fat required no vitamin C supplementation to contain scurvy, despite an almost complete lack of fruit and vegetables.

Should you be worried about nitrates in bacon? The original study has been debunked. Check out http://bit.ly/DontFearBacon we have nitrites in our saliva and celery has lots of it. If a meat is cured with celery powder apparently it can claim to be nitrate free despite possibly having higher levels of nitrate than a standard product.

Two of the richest sources of nitrates (NO3), greater than in bacon, are beetroot juice and celery. It is also frequently found in water. This nitrate is converted by bacteria in saliva to nitrites (NO2) and goes on to help in production of nitric oxide known to reduce blood pressure by dilating small blood vessels in extremities. But don't use mouthwash as this kills the bacteria that do the conversion. Heating nitrates to high heat can cause nitrosamines which may be harmful.

I supplement magnesium, zinc and vitamin K2. Magnesium is important for many functions including bone health and good sleep, while vitamin K2 is unique in its ability to release calcium from arteries where it hardens artery walls and move it into bones where you need it. See next chapter. A Coronary Artery Calcium (CAC) test which measures calcium in artery walls is apparently a good heart attack risk indicator.

CoQ10 is a vitamin like substance found in virtually every cell in the body with the greatest concentrations in the heart. When this level falls, so does general health. CoQ10 is used in the energy producing metabolic pathways of every cell, is a powerful anti-oxidant and without this our bodies cannot survive. An alarming side effect of Statin drugs is the severe depletion of CoQ10 because the body process that the statin interferes with to reduce cholesterol, is part of the same mechanism that produces CoQ10.

What about anti-oxidant supplements? Nick Lane in his very technical book about mitochondria, 'Power sex and suicide' contends that antioxidant supplements have no measurable impact on health and ageing, despite all the marketing hype. He believes that athletes who consume huge amounts of oxygen compared with non-athletes do not generally age more quickly than the average person despite the additional oxygen.

Testing of antioxidant supplements has resulted in very mixed results. This study:

(https://doi.org/10.1016/j.amjcard.2008.02.003) came to the following conclusion:

"Antioxidant therapies have been evaluated in placebo-controlled trials involving tens of thousands of patients. Despite pathophysiologic, epidemiologic, and mechanistic data suggesting otherwise, these clinical trial results have been, to date, mostly negative in the setting of chronic preventative therapy."

The best supplement I absorb is plenty of sunlight which helps the body produce vitamin D from cholesterol.

This study :

(https://pubmed.ncbi.nlm.nih.gov/32918215/) found the following:

"Data support the hypothesis that low sun exposure habits are a major risk factor for all-cause mortality. Low sun exposure is related to an increased risk of death due to CVD and noncancer/non-CVD, and a minor reduction in risk of cancer."

IS "GRASS FINISHED" BETTER?

Who would have thought that moving beef cattle to factory farms, even if only for "finishing", could have such a serious impact on the health of your arteries and your bones. So much so that your level of bodily stiffness, cardio vascular disease risk, arthritis, osteoporosis risk and stroke risk are increased dramatically.

Let me explain how this happens.

When green grass and other green plants use sunlight and photosynthesis to produce energy, they also produce beta-carotene and Vitamin K1. Vitamin K1 (Phylloquinone) was identified in the early 1930's and is important for blood clotting. Most people get plenty of this from eating greens and because the body recycles it, thereby maintaining healthy supplies.

When cows eat green grass, they ingest the Vitamin K1 and then they have the ability to synthesize Vitamin K2 from the K1. Humans are not able to do this in any meaningful quantity and so must get their Vitamin K2 (Menaquinone) from their diet. Good sources include meat, cheese and egg yolks. Perhaps humans lost this ability due to an ancestral diet that was predominantly animal based and therefore provided dietary

Vitamin K2 regularly.

There is an excellent vegetarian source from a Japanese delicacy called natto, which is made from fermented soy in which the introduced bacteria make Vitamin K2.   However, I hear that with its slimy consistency and unpleasant smell, it can be hard to eat.

Vitamin K2 was only identified in the 1970's when it was realized that it had totally different actions within the body. Weston A. Price had identified much earlier that something like it must exist as he had found something extra in traditional diets that was contributing to healthy teeth and jaw development which he called it activator X.

In 1975, The Harvard Medical School discovered that the osteocalcin proteins, which are critical for driving calcium into bones and teeth, were dependent for activation on Vitamin K2. Osteocalcin is the major non-collagen protein found in bone. When activated by Vitamin K2, osteocalcin is converted to a carboxylated protein which can then bind to calcium and this is what the body uses to build teeth and bone. Activated osteocalcin binds free-floating calcium in the blood and transports and integrates it into the bone matrix. So if there is no Vitamin K2, (plus vitamin D) then all the calcium supplements in the world will not build stronger bones or teeth.

So what happens to the calcium if the level of Vitamin K2 is low? Without Vitamin K2 calcium finds other places to build up in tissues within your body with the most critical one being your arteries. You may have heard of hardening of the arteries and this one mechanism that does it. One of the best tests for cardiovascular disease (CVD) is a coronary artery calcium (CAC) scan which measures the level of calcium build up in your arteries. Unlike cholesterol, this measure seems to directly correlate with the risk of cardiovascular disease.

The statistics showing that more than half the

people admitted to hospital for Cardio Vascular Disease (CVD) have normal or low cholesterol levels shows that your CVD risk has little relationship to your cholesterol level. (https://doi.org/10.1016/j.amjcard.2013.05.050), (https://www.uclahealth.org/news/most-heart-attack-patients-cholesterol-levels-did-not-indicate-cardiac-risk).

As you can see, your level of Vitamin K2 is very important for your heart disease risk. Alarmingly, only in 1975 were the very low levels of Vitamin K2 in overall western diets identified, and surprisingly not much is being done about it. Perhaps the problem is just inconvenient, because here is a major problem that is keeping levels very low. If a cow is taken off grass and moved to a concentrated animal feeding operation (CAFO) for its final fattening up prior to becoming food, it is usually fed corn. This is fattening and is low cost due to US government subsidies, so is a most profitable feed for the factory.

Corn has zero Vitamin K1 so the cows body is forced to stop making Vitamin K2. After a short period on corn based feed the cow's level of Vitamin K2 has plummeted to a very low level. Just eyeballing a cow carcass from a CAFO shows much whiter fat which is currently considered desirable in meat on the table. In comparison a grass-fed carcass has a more yellow coloured fat due to the beta-carotene in the grass it has been eating and this also signals a higher level of Vitamin K2. This beta-carotene is the same substance that makes healthy butter yellow, carrots orange and egg yolks orange.

Not only are factory cattle farms implicated in this health disaster, but also eggs. When chickens are fed corn without access to any green vegetable matter or proteins in the form of grubs, worms, insects, etc, their eggs cease to have adequate levels of Vitamin K2. Unfortunately, the old method of using the color of the yolks to verify egg quality is not reliable. Farmers can add chemicals to chicken food to make the yolks more orange.

There is also a, perhaps even more, critical function of Vitamin K2. Not only does it activate calcium so that it can be used to build and repair bone and teeth, reducing the risk of bone fracture, osteoporosis and cavities, but it also activates another protein called "Matrix Gla Protein" (MGP) that removes calcium build up from soft tissues, gradually restoring arteries to their former suppleness. This may reduce blood pressure and may help remove small calcified plaques that might be just starting in your arteries. Animal studies have shown that Vitamin K2 supplementation can produce dramatic reductions in arterial calcium in just 6 weeks. The relationships among Vitamin K2, MGP and arterial calcification are well-established. Studies show that high levels of non-activated MGP are correlated with lower vitamin K2 intake and lower survival rates among cardiovascular patients. (https://doi.org/10.1111/j.1365-2796.2010.02264.x)

Based on this information we should be leveraging the action of Vitamin K2, but most people do not know about these health benefits. Doctors often don't know this and are guilty of putting people on calcium supplements which, without Vitamin K2 plus adequate Vitamin D, are likely to be making arteries harder, increasing the risk of cardiovascular disease while doing nothing to assist with bone density and osteoporosis risk. (https://doi.org/10.1136/bmj.d2040)

Many "health" publications about the value of calcium and vitamin D for bone health, overlook this very critical Vitamin K2 piece of information despite it being known now for many years. This perhaps indicates an article published without full knowledge of the way in which calcium works.

Can Vitamin K2 supplements help. Yes. But a little knowledge is necessary. Vitamin K2 comes in a few forms with the most common being MK4 and MK7. Firstly Vitamin

K2 (Menaquinone) is fat soluble, so you must take these supplements with fat or they will be wasted. This is one of the benefits of eating good quality animal fats, they come with vitamins A,D, E and K2 prepackaged. Secondly if the vitamin is not labelled as K2 them it is probably K1 and this is likely to be of little value to you as it has a very different function in your body.

Menaquinone-4 or MK4 is synthetic Vitamin K2 and has an extremely short half-life. It only lasts a few hours in the body before it is broken down and loses any benefit. If dosing on this it is necessary to take it multiple times during the day. I read that 45 milligrams is the recommended dose.

Menaquinone-7 or MK7 is natural Vitamin K2 and made from natto. This has a half-life of a few days, so a single dose per day is adequate. I read that 120 micrograms or more is the recommended dose. Can you overdose? Apparently not.

If you are on blood thinners for any reason speak to your doctor before taking any of these supplements.

For Vitamin K2 to work it must be paired with adequate levels of both Vitamin D and Vitamin A. These 3 vitamins are only available from the fat of animal foods. You may be surprised by this but in the USA, foods containing beta-carotene are allowed by law to claim they provide vitamin A.

This is not actually correct and your body must convert beta-carotene to vitamin A before it becomes available. Unfortunately this conversion is not efficient in humans (up to 48 molecules for 1 being required) which means that nutrition information labels can be hugely optimistic for the real amount of Vitamin A produced. Compounding this, the absorption rate of beta-carotene can be as low as 20% plus the conversion rate declines as the amount of beta-carotene increases. (https://doi.org/10.1016/s0140-6736(95)92111-7)

The scientific name for Vitamin A is retinol as it was first identified as necessary for vision, with the early signs of Vitamin A deficiency being poor vision in dim light.

Vitamin D as you probably know can also be made in the body from cholesterol when you get adequate sunshine. A research project in 2007 found that Vitamin D supplementation may also be a major factor in reduction of cancer risk for women. (https://doi.org/10.1093/ajcn/85.6.1586)

I read that Vitamin K2 has other benefits such as reducing wrinkles, reducing the impact of Alzheimer's disease, slowing aging, and may assist with Arthritis. Researchers have identified an important inverse relationship between the level of ingested Vitamin K2 and the risk of developing Cancer and death from Cancer. In other words, more Vitamin K2 means a lower risk of Cancer. (https://doi.org/10.3945/ajcn.2009.28691)

URIC ACID

In 1876, Alfred Garrod (1819–1917) identified a link between uric acid and gout. More recent research about uric acid identifies rising levels and suggests that it may more causative in the development of metabolic disease than realized previously. In other words high uric acid levels may directly activate insulin resistance leading to high blood pressure, cardio vascular disease, type-2 diabetes, Alzheimer's, dementia, kidney disease, etc. Who knew?

This study highlights the leading dietary causes of elevated uric acid according to the following relative risk scale: (1.00 = no change, over 1.00 and up = more risk, less than 1.00 and below, possible benefit)
Alcohol = 2.06; Fructose = 1.85; seafood = 1.47; some meats = 1.24; High Purine vegetables = 1.10; Coffee for women = 1.58; Coffee for Men = 0.76; Dairy products = 0.50)

(https://doi.org/10.6133/apjcn.201811_27(6).0022)

Highest risks come from Alcohol and Fructose, (beer has both), with the lowest risks coming from dairy food. (High purine vegetables include: Asparagus, dried beans (especially fava, mung, soy and garbanzo), mushrooms, peas, spinach). (High purine meats were primarily organ meats.) Traditional dietary advice about eating to minimize uric acid often seems to ignore fructose.

The above study suggests that after alcohol, fructose is the biggest danger for raising the risk of uric acid. This leads us to a new awareness that regular drinking of sugar sweetened beverages, energy drinks and sports drinks is akin to ingesting liquid sugar and the uric acid produced may become a major player in the development of metabolic syndrome leading to Type-2 Diabetes, Hypertension, Obesity, Cancer, Kidney disease, Alzheimer's disease and Heart Disease.

The traditional focus on uric acid coming from purines alone, leads to the following type of confusing dietary advice from different health sources:

1. *Apples have a high dietary fiber content which helps in lowering uric acid levels. Fibre absorbs uric acid from the bloodstream and eliminates the excess uric acid from your body.*

2. *The fructose amount stimulates uric acid productio leading to worse consequences. Apples too are a storehouse of natural fructose. Too much consumption of apples can worsen the gout condition even more.*

Check out the following research studies:

Uric acid & fructose: potential biological mechanisms - https://doi.org/10.1016/j.semnephrol.2011.08.006

A causal role for uric acid in fructose-induced metabolic syndrome - https://doi.org/10.1152/ajprenal.00140.2005

The quantity of uric acid becomes the problem with women more at risk after menopause. A human can manage about 5gm of uric acid per day, which is about one apple, so an apple is not a problem, but juicing those apples or any fruit and the total quantity of fruit, and therefore fructose goes way up.

A glass of orange juice has an almost identical nutrition profile to a glass of cola.

An apple a day keeps the doctor away but, 5 apples a day and the doctor you will pay.

FASTING OR (TIME RESTRICTED EATING)

Fasting has become very fashionable and here is why. For years we learned that if we restrict eating, our bodies will cannibalize muscle tissue in its quest for protein, making us lose condition and waste away. But recently we have come to realize that if we do this correctly, not only do we save our muscles, but additionally we get health benefits. Just reducing calories is the wrong way, and will result in hunger, reduction of metabolism, and reduced health.

We have to manage fasting in a way that does not make the body think you are about to be starved. To achieve this, you must first train your body to fuel on fat, becoming metabolically flexible, and then manage the timing of your eating to specific eating windows. A suggested approach is to do intermittent fasting (IF). One of the most common ways to do intermittent fasting, and my particular approach, is to stop eating after dinner, say about 7pm each evening, and not to eat again or snack until the next day at lunch time. This can mean an interval of about 17-18 hours with no eating, followed then by 6 hour eating window.

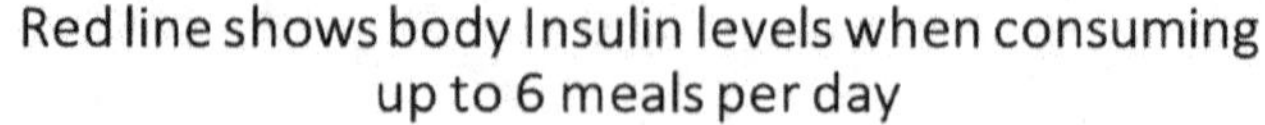

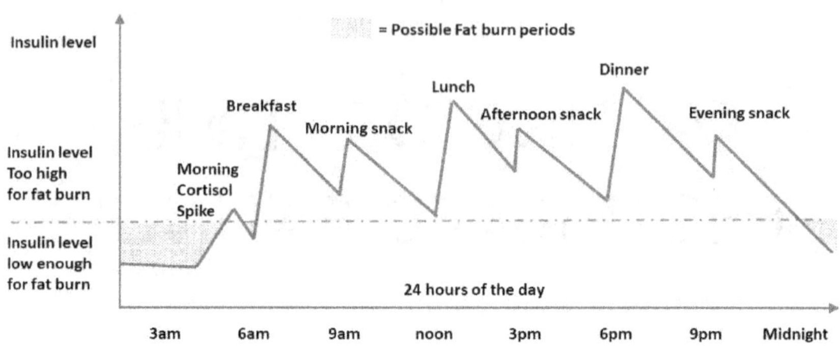

Let's examine why this would be healthy. This long daily interval without eating, and with absolutely no snacking, allows your body to use up the circulating glucose, insulin levels then go low, the body switches to fat burning and uses stored body fat as energy. This can reduce weight, reduce inflammation, lower insulin levels and help your body to become metabolically flexible. If you are 'fat-adapted' then there is generally no feeling of hunger even if the overall dietary calorie level has been reduced. Apparently, this can also trigger rebuilding, repair and housekeeping processes (known as autophagy) within your body which are very beneficial to your overall health. I periodically fast for 24 hours with no hunger at all. Do your own research as there are many approaches to fasting.

It is important to realize that I am not suggesting you eat less then usual, just control when you eat. However, eating a little less is mandatory if fat-loss is your goal.

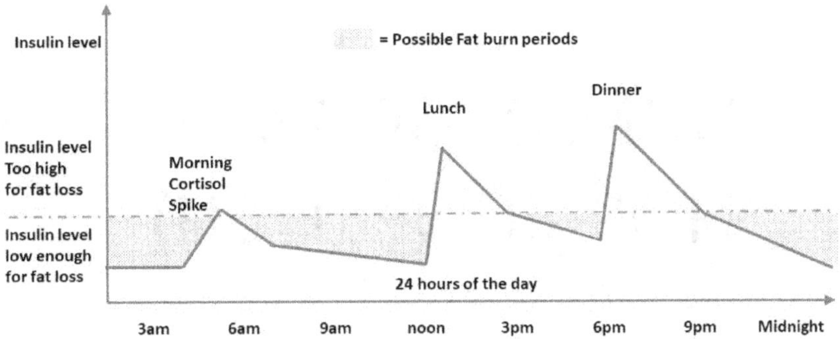

Just in case you are worried about not eating for 18 hours, the world record for fasting is 382 days by a Scotsman, Angus Barbieri. Beginning in June 1965, and with medical supervision he reduced his body weight by 125 kilos. All he consumed was water, tea, coffee and some electrolytes daily. His body was fuelled by his own stored body fat for the whole time.

HUMAN GROWTH HORMONE (HGH)

Human Growth Hormone (HGH) is the stuff that promotes growth in children and the bioavailability of this declines with age. Some body builders and athletes inject this to help build muscles. Fasting can activate about 3 times the level of this hormone naturally, and so it is highly recommended especially for people 50+ to help with bone growth, hair growth, muscle repair, areas all over the body where growth can help to combat ageing.

Human Growth Hormone is a critical hormone for all stages of your life, helping maintain a youthful physique and well-being. It is produced by the pituitary gland, is higher in children and during growth spurts but declines as we age. There are natural ways to increase this but direct supplementation is not recommended. Exercise and good sleep are both critical to getting adequate levels and intermittent fasting (IF) helps. When low, it can result in problems such as loss of energy, increased wrinkles and loss of skin elasticity, reduced muscle mass, and increased depression risk.

A short intense burst of exercise where you sweat and feel the burn will stimulate HGH production, but the levels quickly decline within an hour, suggesting that multiple exercise events during the day may be the most productive.

If you suffer from joint pain, muscle weakness, arthritis, or have diabetes, then more frequent HGH stimulation could be beneficial. Our predominantly high-carbohydrate diet switches off the production of HGH, and any beneficial HGH produced by short intense exercise is negated completely by carb loading immediately before following the exercise. So that energy drink at the gym, with a high carb (sugar) load will depress the HGH driven muscle building activity you may have just stimulated.

HGH is produced in bursts during the day depending on activity with the highest amount released about 30 minutes after you have gone to sleep. During sleep your body mends and builds with the HGH driving growth, strength, muscle building etc. However, if you have just eaten in the 3 hour window prior to bed, you will stimulate insulin release, which reduces this HGH surge.

Dietary sugars, starchy foods and carbohydrates rapidly become glucose in your blood, and any amount above a teaspoonful is toxic, so your body releases the hormone insulin which instructs cells to use or take up this excess glucose to eliminate it. The insulin also suppresses the secretion of Human Growth Hormone (HGH). This means that if you eat immediately before exercise then your body will release insulin which will also suppress the resulting HGH level, so keep the (water) hydration up but avoid the tendency to eat immediately prior to exercise. Protein, water or fats, do not stimulate insulin to the same extent as carbohydrates, fruit and sugar, so can provide the energy and amino acids for muscle building and recovery without driving down HGH levels.

A ketogenic diet where carbohydrates are kept below about 50 grams per day naturally helps ensure HGH availability, because of its ability to keep glucose and therefore insulin levels stable and low.

AUTOPHAGY

In 2017 Yoshinori Ohsum received the Nobel Prize in medicine for his work on improving our understanding of autophagy.

Autophagy is the process by which the body rounds up damaged cells, misfolded proteins and old components and removes or recycles them. In Alzheimer's disease for example, it is believed that these waste components can accelerate the development of the disease. Any way to assist this cleaning process is considered beneficial.

A gerontology researcher, Valter Longo, subjected two different groups of rats to high dose chemotherapy where one group had first been fasted for a period. Over the course of the trial, all the control group rats died, while the fasted group continued to remain healthy. The fasted group had more easily managed the stress of the chemotherapy. Fasting for over 16 hours is an accepted way to kick start autophagy.

In a recent interview with Gabor Erdosi, (A molecular biologist and the brains behind the Facebook group 'Lower Insulin') it was suggested that much of today's western diseases might be related to the absence of any opportunities for autophagy over many years, due to the continuous supply of glucose keeping insulin elevated. This is apparently untested, but maybe the lack of autophagy may not be good for the body in general.

My research suggests that autophagy, which can only occur when insulin is low, has had positive results in treating a wide range of 'diseases of civilisation' particularly heart diseases, brain diseases and 'leaky gut' diseases.

Dr Jason Fung, a Canadian doctor and strong proponent of fasting and autophagy, was asked about the ability of autophagy to assist in the reduction of saggy skin following weight reduction. His answer was that he had no personal experience of a case where a person using fasting and autophagy in the pursuit of weight reduction, also needed to have skin reduction surgery.   Apparently the skin regeneration process can recycle excess collagen, connective tissue and skin left excess due to the volume reduction, gradually eating up skin sag.

The Glucose Ketone Index (GKI) is one way of easily determining the ratio of glucose to ketones in your blood. I have read that the best GKI ratio for autophagy, when targeting cancer or seizures, is under 4, and closer to 1 is better.

For example:

Glucose 5.5 mmol/L;
Ketones 1.5 mmol/L,
Resulting GKI = 5.5/1.5 = 3.7

BENEFITS FOR YOUR BRAIN

The autopsy of Alzheimer diseased brains reveals sticky synapse-destroying plaques made of a protein called amyloid-beta. After insulin molecules do their job and lower the glucose, the body must de-grade the insulin in order to prevent the blood glucose from dropping too low. It does this via an enzyme called insulin-degrading enzyme (IDE). But this enzyme also cleans up amyloid-beta (amyloid) and it is thought that if it is too busy degrading insulin, it may not get to clean up the amyloid. Amyloid is believed to be produced in a normal repair cycle within the brain as part of repair and rebuild activity.

Insulin also binds to the insulin receptor and triggers signalling that supports neuronal survival, but this survival signal is blunted by chronically high insulin levels. As a result of this signalling, insulin resistance is considered by some to be the single most important metabolic contributor to Alzheimer's disease development and progression. This is particularly relevant for women because two-thirds of Alzheimer patients are female.

ReCODE, a program for halting the progression of Alzheimer's disease developed by Dale E. Bredesen MD and credited as being the first treatment to achieve this, identifies as their first intervention, the need to lower insulin via a low carbohydrate Keto diet.

Mild ketosis, it turns out, is optimal for cognitive function: beta-hydroxybutyrate (the most abundant ketone) increases production of the important neuron and synapse supporting molecule BDNF (brain-derived neurotrophic factor), among other effects. There is also a direct relationship showing that people with depression or anxiety have lower levels of BDNF, an important brain growth hormone, in their hippo-campus.

In the study titled 'HbA1c, diabetes and cognitive decline: the English Longitudinal Study of Ageing', of 5189 participants, researchers found 'Significant longitudinal associations between HbA1c levels, diabetes status and long-term cognitive decline'. In other words, higher blood sugar levels were related to long term reduction in brain function.

The ketogenic diet is now a proven therapy for drug resistant epilepsy. Apparently, it has high success when used to treat seizures, particularly in children and has shown promise for treating Parkinson's disease, depression, migraines, and brain cancers.

There is a group of people, including doctors, finding that some people with Alzheimer's disease respond extremely well to high levels of coconut oil or MCT oil in their diet. Not everyone benefits, and introduction must be done slowly to avoid diarrhoea, but results can include a significant return of independence in day-to-day activities such as dressing and eating.

Apparently, a problem related to Alzheimer's is that the brain becomes starved of energy by some problem that denies it access to glucose. The coconut oil or MCT oil provides the brain with ketones which it can use instead of glucose and this can be very beneficial short term. The treatment must be continued daily to maintain the benefit. Coconut oil is mostly saturated fat.

CANCER AND DIET

There is a debate about cancer, as to whether cancer is a genetic disease, i.e. it's in your genes and there is little you can do, or is it a metabolic disease, caused by what you eat, how you live, etc. The metabolic school of thought seems to be leading the argument and this suggests that you have more control over your fate regarding cancer than previously thought.

Do vegetarians suffer less from cancer? It is my understanding that many Hindus in India are strictly vegetarian. They suffer from Cancer as do other vegetarian societies. In the Masai, The Inuit and native Americans on the Great Plains, cancer was rare to absent and these societies were heavy meat eaters, sometimes solely for many months of the year. Although this is only an association, it does seem significant.

In 2007, the World Cancer Research Fund and the American Institute of Cancer Research jointly published a five-hundred-page report entitled 'Food, Nutrition, Physical Activity and the Prevention of Cancer'. The report discusses the evidence linking diet to cancer and finds that the most convincing link is 'greater body fatness' to 'cancers of the colorectal, oesophagus (adenocarcinoma), pancreas, kidney and breast cancer,' and possibly gallbladder cancer as well.

Most significant is that there is a group of 'diseases' including: Type-2 Diabetes Cardio vascular disease (CVD), PCOS, caries, macular degeneration, obesity, hypertension, stroke, Alzheimer's and Cancer. These diseases are sometimes referred to as 'Western' diseases as their prevalence significantly increases after a society adopts western style nutrition including sugar, white flour and polyunsaturated seed oils. So, although we don't hear it stated, cancer growth does seem to be assisted by the standard low fat, high carb diet including polyunsaturated seed oils.

Most cancer cells feed on glucose, some on glutamine. While normal cells can live on ketones and fats, most cancer cells are unable to do this, instead glycolysis or breakdown of glucose is their only food. German scientist Otto Warburg identified this over 90 years ago and in 1931 was awarded the Nobel prize for this work. (https://doi.org/10.1016/j.tibs.2015.12.001)

When speaking to an oncologist about this he suggested that this was a myth. However, proof of this is the process for a Positron Emission Tomography (PET) scan. For this the patient is injected with a radioactive tracer. The scan then highlights the places in the body where the radioactive tracer has accumulated. The radio-tracer is a radioactive sugar. The one commonly used is called FDG (fluorodeoxyglucose). Cancer cells are very active when they are growing and reproducing in a specific area. They need energy to grow. So, active cancer cells take up the FDG which then shows up brighter on the scan.

This highlights a new direction that cancer treatment is taking to deprive cancer of its energy source by restricting glucose while hitting it with various treatments.

Researchers have found that higher insulin and glucose levels make cancer less sensitivity to chemotherapy. With a Keto diet, chemotherapy is apparently more effective, cancer is more sensitive to the treatment and patients can expect a faster and easier recovery. There is a recommendation that they should also fast for 3 days prior to chemo, fast during the chemo and then for 2 days following. This comes from Dr Nashua Winters and Valter D. Longo, but undertake your own research of course. From Annette Bosworth MD comes the information that one of the most renowned cancer treatment centers in the world, M. D. Anderson in Texas USA, will not begin chemotherapy for brain cancer until the patient has been in ketosis for 2 weeks.

There is a secondary related effect of high levels of Insulin Like Growth Factor (IGF-1) caused by high levels of insulin, stimulating cancer growth. Both have been known about for decades but largely ignored by mainstream cancer therapy. This suggests that a low carbohydrate diet, reducing glucose in the body and thereby lowering insulin levels, could halt or slow cancer proliferation.

Professor Jurgen Schole, from the University of Hanover, in 1986 after his low carbohydrate research said, *"we were able to demonstrate that the rates of tumour growth in experimental animals, which follow the application of carcinogens, diminish significantly when carbohydrates are replaced by the isocaloric amount (same calorific value) of fat."*

The adulteration of normal cells to pre-cancerous cells happens continuously in your body as cells and their mitochondria are damaged by regular low-level insults. Examples include smoke, chemicals, pollution, radiation, asbestos, excess sugar, oxidized food substances, and inflammation. Killer T-cells seek out these damaged cells and kill them before they can proliferate. Support your immune system to maintain this protection. Below are some steps to assist you to maintain a healthy and active immune system:
1. Eat real food, meat, eggs, fish, vegetables, avoid refined carbohydrates, sugars, starches.

2. Use natural oils, animal fats, olive, coconut, avocado oil, avoid all seed (vegetable) oils.
3. Exercise regularly then rest and recover.
4. Get good sleep with a regular wake up time.
5. Avoid alcohol and sugar substitutes.
6. Adopt time restricted eating, perhaps 16:8. No snacking, 2 meals per day.
7. Get regular sunlight on your skin, without burning.

As already mentioned, the repeated heating and cooling of Omega-6 polyunsaturated oils in restaurant fryers, breaks down molecules, oxidizing the oils and creating new compounds and this gets worse as the heating is repeated, and it contaminates and reduces the 'smoke point' for the oil. Novel polymers are produced, that cause problems for restaurant cleaning, with new and more powerful cleaning compounds needed to remove the residues from walls and drains.

If we work in these fumes, or eat food cooked in this 'soup', I am not surprised that cancer rates are rising. At home you can avoid this by frying in saturated fat with lard, tallow, avocado oil, butter or coconut oil.

I am aware of a suggestion, that long term use of 'fat soluble' statins is anecdotally linked to multiple cancer events in people, maybe because the statin mechanism is to interrupt the body's manufacture of LDL cholesterol, which itself is considered a healing material and integral to an immune response.

If you want additional information about surviving cancer and using diet to increase the effectiveness of current cancer therapy I suggest the following excellent book:
"How to starve Cancer" by Jane McLelland
Her website at: https://www.howtostarvecancer.com

SO WHY DO DIETS OFTEN FAIL?

If in order to lose weight, you choose to eat less calories each day than your body needs, then because your body is always trying to maintain a state of balance, it gradually reduces your metabolism to try and match the lowered incoming energy level. To do this it reduces the energy available to do less critical things such as, maintain your body, keep you warm, undertake bone repair, grow healthy hair, fuel muscle growth, and it gradually cuts down these body functions to ensure that the core functions continue to operate to keep you alive. In addition, it sends urgent messages to your brain, that you are hungry.

If this condition becomes unbearable and you once again resume eating at previous levels, the lower metabolism level is quickly satiated but you are now consuming surplus food. This surplus is stored as fat and the result is that you quickly gain back the weight lost plus more, until your metabolism gradually recovers to the new food level. This metabolism recovery can apparently take years, with some of 'The Biggest Looser' contestants taking up to 6 years to repair their damaged metabolism.

There is a solution to this problem which is to become metabolically flexible. If you train your body to operate on fats instead of sugars and glucose, and continue to eat this way, then when you reduce your food level, your body will begin burning the body fat you saved up when you had excess energy. The difference is that the energy obtained from the stored fat prevents your body from believing it is going into starvation. When your body operates on fats, your food triggers satiation sensors which means that despite eating less, you do not feel hungry.

It takes anything from 3 days to 3 weeks to get the body used to this change (fat-adapted) and in the interim period some people get uncomfortable flu like symptoms. Eventually these go away and you become 'metabolically flexible', meaning that you are able to feed your body on fats or glucose (sugars), whichever is available. This also means that you lose your insulin resistance, becoming insulin sensitive, returning your body to correct functioning.

It is worth mentioning that a change like this should not be seen as a diet to be used for a short time and then you revert to your previous eating patterns. Going Keto or Paleo is a lifestyle change. In my case I expect to be on Keto forever unless I learn that there is some critical aspect to it that endangers my health.

HOW ABOUT A BALANCED DIET

Is balance good? What should we balance? You should not be balancing macronutrients in a meal when eating, because if there are high or even medium levels of carbohydrates in every meal, then your body will always have plenty of insulin available and fat will always be stored and never released from your fat storage. The concept of a balanced diet is meaningless.

Instead, any balancing needs to be about balancing higher levels of dietary carbohydrates with very low carbohydrates each day. A number of the meals you eat, should have very low carbohydrates so that your stored fats can be utilised and satiety switches activated. This would enable your body to get a sustained period daily when insulin is low and fats can be released from storage for energy.

FERTILITY

Human fertility seems to be declining. My research suggests that there are dietary ways to assist with this problem and increase fertility.

A female body will be reluctant to get pregnant if there are signs that the environment is not suitable to sustain a baby. How could it establish this?

One clear way to determine a good environment is the dietary nutrition level. This could be due to the external conditions or could be due to the food choices being made. Studies referenced below suggest that a low level of critical nutrients such as folate, vitamin K2, carnitine, vitamin B12, taurine, zinc and riboflavin may influence the ability to conceive.

The role of anti-oxidants in our diet and also those produced in the body is to reduce oxidative stress caused by the action of free radicals. Dietary anti-oxidants may benefit, but apparently the most important anti-oxidant is glutathione. This is produced in the body and depends on the availability of some critical nutrients and molecules for its production. With low levels of this, the body can suffer from higher oxidative stress which may also signal an unsuitable environment for a baby. My understanding is that a high level of PUFA (Omega-6) seed oils in the diet has proven to drive up oxidative stress.

The level of insulin in the body could also be a factor, particularly because the ovaries apparently never become insulin resistant like other organs. Most women with PCOS (Polycystic Ovary Syndrome) also have a high level of insulin. Insulin is increased by a diet that is heavy in sugars and carbohydrates and seems to have a direct impact on the hormone balance during the ovulation cycle.

In a normal situation the release of an egg from the follicles in the ovaries is triggered by a spike in a hormone called luteinizing hormone. In a woman with PCOS, the ovaries make additional testosterone which drives some additional hair growth, dark skin patches and acne problems, plus the level of luteinizing hormone is much higher. It seems that this prevents the normal ovulation spike of this hormone, and an egg is not released. This failure of the normal mechanism can apparently be a cause of irregular menstruation.

It is not clear if the higher insulin level causes PCOS or these are concurrent conditions however lowering insulin levels through diet seems to help. I have read of woman who have failed to get pregnant despite multiple IVF treatments, who become pregnant after a period of 2-3 months on a low carbohydrate diet.

This study https://doi.org/10.1210/jendso/bvad112
"The effects of Ketogenic Diet on Reproductive Hormones in Women with Polycystic Ovary Syndrome" found that Short-term ketogenic diet potentially improved hormonal imbalances commonly associated with PCOS.

Males are not exempt from these impacts as well. Erectile disfunction (ED) is one symptom of excess insulin in the body. Again, this can be a result of a diet that is high in sugars and carbohydrates and can also be impacted by the habit of snacking all day. Regular snacking including sugary drinks, prevents the body from achieving a regular period of low insulin when other functions such as autophagy can occur. If you are male and never wake with an erection then you should see this as a warning sign.

Nutrition can also impact male fertility with a report outlined below which links a low level of taurine with lower male fertility. Taurine is usually obtained from the meat, shellfish, chicken, tuna or dairy in your diet.

https://www.ncbi.nlm.nih.gov/pmc/articles/PMC6480978/ or
https://www.ncbi.nlm.nih.gov/pmc/articles/PMC5904600/ or
https://www.sciencedaily.com/
releases/2018/05/180511102357.htm

DOES EXERCISE HELP?

You may have realized by now that getting fat is not about calories in and calories out, but about the type of calories you are eating, although eating too much will keep you fat.   If you are choosing to use this type of lifestyle for weight loss then you will need to eat a little less than you may have eaten previously. However, the low carbohydrate, higher fat and intermittent fasting approach makes this very sustainable. I have now been living this way since 2019 and enjoy my meals more than I ever used to.

Does exercise help? Watch the entrants at the local fun-run, and you will see plenty of people who are doing aerobic exercise regularly but who are not particularly slim.

In 1989 a team of Danish researchers published the results of a trial whereby they trained a group of 18 sedentary men and 9 sedentary women for 18 months to compete in a marathon. After the marathon the men had on average lost 5 pounds of body fat and the women had lost zero. Their conclusion, 'no change in body composition was observed'. Dr Timothy Noakes says *"if you have
to exercise to control your weight, then your diet is wrong"*

Testing has shown that exercise increases your appetite and the net result of exercise is little to zero benefit for weight loss. It is good to help with general health, building blood cells, body composition and flexibility. Exercise, particularly resistance training, such as weight lifting does use food energy and will deplete glucose from muscles which does reduce the amount to be stored as fat, but the overall result is insignificant, compared with a change in diet.

Going for a brisk walk immediately after a meal is one sure way to help reduce glucose levels.

Building muscle with resistance training can be particularly beneficial for older people, many of whom become incapacitated in later life due to a fall or balance problem, indirectly caused by loss of their muscular strength.

Your body stores glucose as glycogen in skeletal muscles, to have energy immediately available for a fight or flight response. Estimates for an average male, 70 grams in the liver and 210 grams in the muscles. Increasing muscle volume or depleting the glycogen stored in the muscles will help with the removal of glucose from your blood and help normalise blood sugar levels, reducing the glucose available for fat storage. Low intensity aerobic exercise is unlikely to help, as the level of energy used is low (slow twitch fibres), however high intensity exercise engages fast twitch muscle fibres depleting higher levels of stored glycogen and so providing additional storage for glucose. (Slow twitch vs fast twitch muscle fibres refer to the rate of fatiguing of the muscle fibre, not speed of contraction).

What about athletic performance? Early testing of endurance athletes on ketogenic diets saw performance reduce when using fat as fuel. Because the time required to become adapted to fat as fuel was not understood, most testing was limited to 3 weeks or less. From this a belief developed that carbohydrate fuelled performance was superior.

Recent testing has shown that once an endurance athlete is fully fat adapted, having maintained a low carb diet for around

3-6 months, athletic performance can be better than previous glucose fuelled levels. In addition, the glycogen levels in muscles is maintained exactly as for a glucose fueled athlete. As a result, a number of athletes are switching to a low carbohydrate diet, however they may not want to advertise this performance advantage.

Although this may not be very applicable to most people, if you are an elite athlete, take a look at this video for further information: https://youtu.be/KF3buYQWJ3E.

According to fat adapted keto athletes, they recover faster following a hard workout. Any exercise will provide greater benefit if it is done during the fasting window of an intermittent fast. This is good in the morning and assists in counteracting the impact of the typical early morning cortisol spike which increases glucose and blunts your response to insulin.

US researchers Dr. Jeff Volek and Dr. Stephen Phinney produced an excellent book on Keto Diets and performance titled: "The Art and Science of Low Carbohydrate Performance" where they recorded and analysed their observations from conducting a number of tests on elite athletes using ketogenic diets.

Cutting calories without the benefit of fat adaption may lead to breakdown of muscle as your body seeks to access sufficient protein. However, once fat adapted your body creates human growth hormone (HGH) during a fast, which preserves muscle by preventing this break down from occurring until your body fat level goes below about 4%. This is a very low-fat level even for extreme athletes. Keeping up your exercise levels will help build and maintain muscles, which is so important to maintaining strength and longevity as you age.

This is a good time to remind the reader that if you choose to reduce calories, do not reduce your protein levels. Keeping protein levels up is generally healthier. You may need to increase protein to compensate for the protein in any carb based food you no longer eat.

For the High Intensity Interval Training (HIIT) follower, it may be beneficial to become metabolically flexible. This means that you can run your body on either glucose or fat and usually requires a period of fat adaption to achieve this. The reason is that a high intensity session can deplete the glycogen from your muscles significantly and if you are then short of glucose, but not fat adapted (Your body cannot fuel from stored fat), the result might be some cannibalization of muscle mass to immediately regenerate the glycogen in the muscles. You could lose some of that muscle you are working so hard to build.

If you experience dizziness, shakes or hunger following a HIIT session, this can be a signal that you are temporarily short of glucose (blood sugar) and not fat adapted.

From my reading of "Body by Science" by Doug McGuff and "Body for Life" by Bill Phillips, I have adopted an exercise routine that should keep me fit and build strength to help balance the gradual loss of muscle as I age.

The principles are: resistance training for strength and health with some aerobic running for balance, flexibility and stamina. Resistance training muscles are worked intensively to failure, over a very short period, in order to engage fast twitch fibres. Because these fibers are very slow to recover you need to allow 4-7 days recovery for any specific muscle group. This resistance training also depletes maximum volumes of glycogen from the muscles helping to deplete glucose as the glycogen is replenished.

Is it working for me? My initial attempts to do chin-ups were pathetic, but now I can complete 15 reps and complete 15 push-ups with a 20Kg weight plate on my back.

Do your own research as I am not a personal trainer.

INFLAMATION

This might be the most important thing you can learn about your health.

When you damage yourself such as with a burn, cut or a splinter, it is sore, the damaged area goes red and sometimes swells up a little. A scab can form over the damaged area and if the offending item is still present, pus can form around it as your body attempts to isolate it and repair. Eventually the pus dissipates, the wound heals, and the redness goes away. This is normal. This is inflammation. Your body is fighting against things that harm it.

When you eat foods that your body is not designed for, or get stressed, or breath toxins in the air and other insults, you introduce into your body, offending items and the response inside you is just the same as above. These offending items cause inflammation and maybe blood clots. When the inflammation is in your arteries, the end result is usually Cardio Vascular Disease (CVD).

Having read this far you now know that cholesterol does not cause heart disease so what is the cause. *"Heart disease is caused by chronic low-grade inflammation"*. Source Dr. Dwight Lundell.

Dr. Dwight Lundell, with experience of 5000 open heart

surgeries, has produced a free pdf book titled *"The Great Cholesterol Lie. Why inflammation kills and the real cure for heart disease"*. It is available for free download here. https://www.scribd.com/document/412364188/ GreatCholesterLie-1 I can thoroughly recommend it.

However as covered earlier, heart disease may be caused by arterial blood clots (thrombus) and explained by the Thrombic Process. See a full explanation in the chapter on cholesterol.

The standard low fat / high carbohydrate diet as promoted by official dietary advice can be pro-inflammatory. Many foods eaten are processed foods with chemicals and additives that your body has never evolved to deal with. As a result, it believes it is under attack and an inflammatory response is triggered. The increased fat storage from the action of excess carbohydrates increases the production of inflammatory compounds in the adipose fat cells. More body fat equals more inflammation.

Sugar is inflammatory, and food allergies are inflammatory. Excess sugar agitates the lining of blood vessels. Dairy and nut allergies can trigger inflammatory responses. The same food toxins in vegetables that fight off the plant's insect attackers are inflammatory within our digestion system and eventually in our blood.

Persistent stress which triggers cortisol and stimulates the fight or flight response is inflammatory because of the same response whereby the body perceives that it is under attack. Persistent high insulin levels are inflammatory as can be hormone imbalances, particularly in women.

The products we have around us that are made from synthetic compounds and the chemicals that leach from these are inflammatory in just the same way that smoking introduces inflammatory particles into our lungs and then into our bloodstream.

We also absorb these compounds through our skin in the same way that a nicotine patch works. This should raise some questions for people putting chemicals on their skin for cosmetic or sunscreen purposes. What is in them? Are they safe? I have read of people on the carnivore diet using refined beef tallow as a moisturiser in order to minimize the impact of chemicals on their skin.

Check out this Reuters Investigation of Johnson and Johnson: (https://www.reuters.com/investigates/special-report/ johnsonandjohnson-cancer/) Imagine finding out that you used baby powder that was contaminated with asbestos. It highlights that some cosmetic companies may not ensure their chemicals are safe.

Polyunsaturated Omega-6 (PUFA) from vegetable oils is inflammatory. Replacing dietary saturated fat with polyunsaturated fat creates inflammation in cells and inflammation in mitochondria. Omega-6 levels in US body fat have risen from 9% in 1961 to 25% in 2003. In women's breast milk over the period 1940-2000 inflammatory omega-6 levels have risen from 6% to 20+%. (Source Dr. Gary Fettke). We not only eat more of this, but we also cook much of our food in these oils and add it as dressings. With low levels of Omega-3 oils which traditionally would balance out the Omega-6 oils, we have created a PUFA imbalance which the body must attempt to deal with.

The ketogenic diet can significantly reduce overall inflammation by controlling a number of mechanisms responsible for raising this. For example, it promotes the production of the ketone, beta-hydroxybutyrate (BHB) which works on inflammation by inhibiting the NLRP3 inflammasome, an inflammatory protein triggered by infections, tissue damage, or metabolic imbalances. BHB has a similar effect in the body as ibuprofen.

The dietary advice outlined in this book shows how you can use food as medicine to address these problems. It all starts with reducing sugar, Omega-6 seed oils, ultra-processed foods (UPF) and carbohydrates.

It may be coincidence, but in Mid-2019 I returned home from overseas with serious back pain, which I had endured for over 6 months. It was identified by an MRI scan as a lower lumbar disk protrusion and I was unable to sit back in the aircraft seats on the trip. I began the keto diet within a week. Three months later I had lost about 5 kg, the chronic pain had gone and I was walking freely. Diet and physiotherapy had addressed the problem without surgery. Maybe the ability of keto to reduce inflammation was material.

SUNSHINE

Should we seek the shade all day or just during the midday sun. Here is what I have come to believe.

For thousands of years humans spent lots of time in sunshine, some with minimal clothing. Our skin pigmentation evolved as we migrated out of Africa, getting more transparent, perhaps, to ensure that we receive more of the benefit from the weaker sun's rays in the higher latitudes. Maybe this is because it is very important for our health.

A few decades ago, we regularly treated some ailments with sun exposure. TB treatment is the most obvious example. It is fascinating that some diseases such as MS correlate with latitude. The further you are from the equator, the higher the risk of Celiac disease, Type 1 diabetes, rheumatoid arthritis, Crohn's disease, lupus, psoriasis and MS. This is from the American MS website: https://mymsaa.org/ms-information/overview/who-gets-ms/

Individuals living beyond the 40-degree mark north or south of the equator are far more likely to develop MS, and this is especially true for people in North America, Europe, and southern Australia

UV rays in sunshine are categorized into UVA with a longer

wavelength and UVB with a shorter wavelength and they are different in the impact they have on the human body.

UVA with its long wavelength is able to penetrate glass, the atmosphere and penetrate deeper into skin. As a result of this it is more responsible for creating a tan as the skin responds to this insult and increases the level of melanin for natural protection. By gradual exposure to this effect , it seems that we may be able to build up a protective layer that will minimize skin damage and possibly protect against skin cancers. I understand that skin cancer risk is very high in office workers and maybe this is due to a lack of regular sun conditioning.

I read that we should not equate skin damage to getting a tan. A tan is not skin damage. Skin damage comes for the intense action of UVB. However, skin damage will most certainly occur whilst getting a tan if the concurrent UVB exposure is high or prolonged.

UVB has a shorter wavelength and is much more dangerous, creating sunburns which can apparently confer life-long cancer risk. Because of its short wavelength, UVB is filtered by the atmosphere and so should be avoided during the middle of the day when it is directly overhead and has less atmosphere to be filtered through. It is suggested that if you are sunbathing for health, then do so when your shadow is longer than your height, because this will be the time that the atmosphere is filtering out most of the harmful UVB rays. Sunburn will cause DNA damage so should be definitely avoided.

With sun exposure your body makes vitamin D from cholesterol and also makes Nitric Oxide (NO).

Many studies have shown that this exposure correlates with higher levels of natural immunity, improves sleep and reduces the risk of many diseases. Surprisingly the same impact of vitamin D has not been able to be duplicated with supplementation, which is perhaps related to this next point. Sun exposure also helps your body create nitric oxide (NO) which is very important for your health. It is critical for blood pressure control and for the blood pumping action of arteries and veins. The little blue pill defeats ED by the action of the nitric oxide it helps create.

A Scandinavian study set out to look at the impact of sun exposure on longevity. They found that on average higher sun exposure people benefited from longer life. See:-

https://pubmed.ncbi.nlm.nih.gov/26992108/ below is part of their conclusion

Nonsmokers who avoided sun exposure had a life expectancy similar to smokers in the highest sun exposure group, indicating that avoidance of sun exposure is a risk factor for death of a similar magnitude as smoking. Compared to the highest sun exposure group, life expectancy of avoiders of sun exposure was reduced by 0.6-2.1 years.

It is puzzling to see the massive growth of skin cancers over the last few decades given the high levels of sun exposure of our ancestors. Is it due to a much greater focus on finding this damage, to lower ozone protection, or is something else at play here? If the increasing levels of skin cancer are compared with the level of polyunsaturated seed oils (PUFA's) in the diet, there is a very close correlation. Maybe this is significant. PUFA's will replace saturated fat in cellular membranes and the level of these fats is growing rapidly in the skin of humans on the standard American diets of today.

A healthy person has about 2% PUFA in their body fat, however many people these days have up to 30% PUFA in their body fat. These polyunsaturated seed oils, have only been part of our diet since 1911, and come as soy bean oil, corn oil, canola, safflower oils, rice bran oil, sunflower oil, etc. They are very prone to oxidation due to the molecular structure and it is believed by some that they can promote oxidation in the whole body.

Cellular membranes are critical to health as they are part of every cell and if compromised by oxidized oils may be accelerating problems such as whole-body inflammation, fatigue, and the risk of cancers. Conversely saturated fats which up until the late 1900's were the most common dietary fats, are very resistant to oxidation due to their hydrogen-saturated molecular structure and lack of double bonds.

Some people who have adopted diets that shun PUFA seed oils, replacing them with saturated fats, are claiming that they suffer from less sunburn, can spend more time outdoors without discomfort and keep their tans for much longer.

Because seed oils have a half-life in the human body of about 2 years, and are endemic in ultra-processed food, restaurant fryers and fast food, it will take a long time for someone to know if this impact is also their experience. This needs to be researched further as it could be much healthier than slathering your skin with dubious (possibly carcinogenic) chemicals in order to reduce UVB sun damage.

Some chemicals and food can make skin more sensitive to sun damage. Lack of vitamin B3 (Niacin or Nicotinamide) and lack of vitamin B12 (Cobalamin) make people more sensitive to sun damage, in fact some believe that B3 can reduce the risk of skin cancer by actively assisting with sun damage repair. Artificial sweeteners, some citrus fruits, figs, parsley, celery, dill, fennel and NSAIDS are reported to increase photosensitivity in human skin for some people.

HOW DO I KEEP HEALTHY THROUGHOUT THIS MESS?

Based on what we have reviewed, if you follow a diet that minimizes processed food, avoids processed carbohydrates like sugar and flour, and drastically reduces (PUFA) Omega-6 oils, you will be healthier than if you are eating a standard (low fat / high carb) diet.

The combination of fructose, refined carbohydrates and polyunsaturated oils creates inflammation in arteries throughout the body. Inflammation of blood vessels is a major trigger for cardio vascular disease (CVD).

There are some diets that can help you take back your health. The Paleo diet, the Keto diet, the carnivore diet and the Low Carb High Fat diet (LCHF). With these diets, your body runs mostly on fatty acids and frequently operates in a state of ketosis where it is using your body fat for its daily energy supply. This has multiple benefits:

- It helps lower insulin which reduces the risk of type 2 diabetes,
- Improves blood markers,
- Helps reduce heart attack risk,
- Helps reduce weight and obesity,
- Reduces risk of other conditions such as fatty liver disease, macular degeneration of eyes, kidney disease and many others plus,
- The PURE study showed that people live longer on a low carbohydrate diet.

What happens on the keto diet or a low carbohydrate high fat (LCHF) diet?

First you try not to eat any processed food, which means when you are in the supermarket you can avoid the middle of the store as that is where most of the processed food and Omega-6 filled products are.

Secondly you read nutrition labels on food packaging and avoid grains and all the seed oils like sunflower oil, soya bean oil, corn oil, canola oil, rice bran oil, etc.

Thirdly you avoid sugar and try to reduce your carbohydrate levels to around 50 grams per day or less.

One of the best things about the Keto or LCHF diet is that as you become a fat-burner, the first fat you burn off is usually the visceral fat that is stored around your middle and your organs. This can result in a smaller waistline measurement and a lowered health risk.

Don't get too concerned about whether you get into ketosis or not, or what your level of ketones actually is. Measurement is unnecessary in my experience and higher ketone levels do not always mean a better result. Ketones are actually the by-product of an incomplete oxidation of fatty acids. You just might be managing a more complete oxidation of these. So long as you find that you are losing inches off your waist measurement and you are not feeling hungry, then you can be sure you are achieving the necessary low glucose / low insulin levels.

As your body becomes more adapted to using ketones for energy, the levels you measure may fall as the ketones are more completely consumed. Don't be concerned if this is happening. The actual ketone level is not that important.

Because a lower level of carbohydrate and insulin in the body allows the kidneys to release more water, I find that I pee a little more, but the benefit of this is that it is a signal to me that I am in ketosis.

A less known side benefit of keto is that the body can shed excess energy when in a state of ketosis by expelling ketones in urine and in breath. Each little parcel of excess energy is 4 calories. This may help reduce excess body fat.

WHAT DOES EATING THIS WAY, MEAN FOR ME?

I nitially I felt I was missing a lot of what I particularly liked because I enjoyed many of the foods that I was now restricting, such as bread, pasta, bagels, cake, cookies, scones, muesli bars, cereals and most factory-made packaged foods. The reduction in sweetness was initially less pleasant, but I found that I adapted very quickly.

It is natural to focus on the foods you are losing, but appreciate for a moment that this is just because they are foods that you have grown up with. If you had been born into a different culture, you would probably have learned to eat very different foods. This change is really just a healthy adjustment from old habits.

If you are struggling with this change, seek support and make the change using friends and family to assist. My wife and I did this together and I believe this made it much easier. However, as you learn what to eat, you will develop new favorites and gradually adapt to the change. Keep in mind that you are doing this for your health which becomes even more important as you age.

So what do I eat more of now? I have found that I eat more eggs, cream, fish, meats, vegetables and what might be called 'real food'. One of the ways to know if a food is good for me is to check it has very little processing. Minimally processed food, or food without a nutrition label is probably best.

If you can handle dairy, then you might eat more cheese and I recommend that you minimize milk and eat more cream. Surprisingly, real cream has less sugar than milk and is less likely to trigger lactose intolerances, plus the additional saturated fat is good for your body.

When it comes to vegetables, I really only avoid two. Potato and Corn. Almost everything else is okay for me, although above ground vegetables generally have lower levels of carbohydrates. I have found that I eat more vegetables than ever before. This diet can also be followed if you are vegetarian or vegan, but you need to make sure you are getting all the nutrition you need.

Meat has huge levels of nutrients, usually more bio-available to your body than vegetable sourced nutrients. Meat can even provide sufficient vitamin C. Getting sufficient vitamin B12, zinc, iron and Omega-3 PUFA is apparently a problem if you don't eat any animal products, particularly for young children as it is critical for brain development. Vitamin B12 deficiency can cause irreversible nervous system degeneration, so is a very serious worry.

One concern I should address is the perception that eating meat increases your risk of cancer. My research suggests this is a myth spread by groups that want to influence you to avoid meat. For confirmation take a look here: https://bit.ly/2oNCYT2.

On a practical note, I would recommend you find some good Keto, low carb or Paleo cookbooks and set about learning some new recipes and cooking skills. There is a good vegetarian book called Keto-tarian for those who want to avoid meat which also highlights how easy it is to fall into becoming an unhealthy 'carbotarian', by eating an almost entirely carbohydrate laden diet. You will find that eating low carb often requires more kitchen preparation as there are far less off-the-shelf foods available at present, however if your experience is like mine, you will find that you enjoy eating much more.

See my special note for vegans later in the book.

At the end of this book are some basic recipes I have found to be useful in the transition.

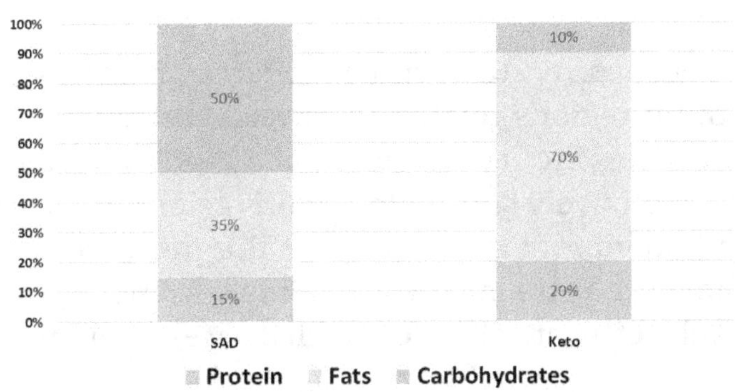

ARE CARBS ADDICTIVE?

Are some carbohydrates addictive? A number of researchers are taking this thought seriously and conducting studies to try and establish the reality of carbohydrate food addictions.

A study published in 2013, titled, "Effects of dietary glycemic index on brain regions related to reward and craving in men", by Lennerz, Alsop, etc, concluded that a high GI meal increased hunger and selectively stimulated brain regions associated with reward and craving in a period after the meal which impacts eating behaviour at the next meal. This was more pronounced when the subjects were obese or carried excess weight.

I have personal experience of children who when consuming specific sugar sweetened drinks would often become very excited and energetic, followed about 1 hour later by a significant drop in mood that often resulted in tears and anger.

There is a recognition that for some people, transitioning to a low carb diet is very difficult as they struggle to give up their favourite carb heavy food, such as pasta or bread. For these people one recommendation is that complete abstinence from the particular food may be the only way to overcome this addiction.

Despite my own transition to a low carb mostly keto diet and maintaining this since 2019, I have found some fascinating things happening in my mind. I think I have always operated this way but it is much more obvious now. For example, if I am at a buffet, and depending on the food, I often find myself looking for the largest piece available. I certainly don't need a large piece but something seems to trigger this desire.

If I look into the refrigerator and see a piece of fruit pie, my senses light up and I start to think about when I could eat it and what I would have with it. If I am cutting a small slice from a bigger cake, despite my chosen low carb guidelines and decision to only have a tiny piece as a treat, I sometimes find myself cutting a larger piece. Do I need it? No! Do I want it? Hell yes. I have learned it is actually easier if the slices are all pre-cut so that I just get to take one slice, or maybe just ask someone else to do the serving. Once my piece is in front of me on the plate, all those feelings seem to vanish.

When I am with a group sharing out the available food, I find myself watching closely what others are taking and have to work quite hard to take a small piece and adhere to the old adage FHB, (Family Hold Back). When I have a cup of tea, I have got into the habit of having a small snack with it during my afternoon eating window. I certainly don't need it but the cuppa does not seem the same without it.

If I am asked "would I like a piece of dark (>72%) chocolate?" Then the answer is almost always yes, even if I have just eaten a large meal. It is almost as if the question gives me permission to cheat on my own eating behaviour guidelines.

Are these symptoms of an addiction. Maybe they are. It is

certainly not great behavior, and makes me very aware of the difficulty some people must have when choosing to give up their favourite foods.

What helps? One thing that helps enormously is to visualise the food as particularly unhealthy and this works very well when I am avoiding the whole food item such as a sweetened beverage, cookie or a donut. However it fails miserably when taking a portion of something that I have already decided is OK in a very small quantity.

The best solution seems to be to avoid the temptation in the first instance. Stay away from that aisle in the supermarket, or avoid that particular shop. Try to ensure that these addictive foods are not in the pantry at home or are well hidden. If the pantry or refrigerator is full of the good stuff, then it becomes easy to select from these items and not succumb to the bad stuff.

Having a few of "George's Crackers" available, based on my cracker recipe in this book is hugely helpful as I can just take 1 or 2 of these and know that this is the good stuff, and I am still sticking to my eating plan. My favourites have salt and cracked black pepper on them.

PLANT BASED DIETS

There is a push, by some, for adoption of plant-based diets, which argues that our herds of meat food herbivores are bad for the environment. This is surprising because herds, such as the North American Buffalo in the past that apparently numbered over 60 million, were located all over the world and the environment was better than today when all of these are now gone. Early COVID19 lock downs resulted in massively improved air quality levels despite the continuation of animal farming. This seems to be another situation where a profit motive by business seems to be driving the agenda, rather than the health of humans.

In the USA, beef cattle contribute to 1.4% of greenhouse gasses.

Water use is an example of the false claims made around animal farming. 94+% of the water used for beef production comes from rain and snow. This is not water that could be used for anything else and is doing what we want it to do. Irrigating the land naturally.

Stated claims about CO2 and methane impacts by grazing animals, have been found to be widely exaggerated and they ignore the fact that animal sourced CO2 and methane is not new, but is cycled continuously whereas the CO2 increasing in the atmosphere is new CO2 coming from fossil fuels.

Most plant food consumed today comes from a small group of plants including, wheat, sugar, potatoes, corn, and rice. Much of this is fertilized by oil industry sourced artificial fertilizers, grown in huge monoculture areas, and subsidized by government, resulting in a very cheap product. This process depletes soils but the resulting grains can be converted into many processed foods and sold at a huge profit.

Even vegetarians and vegans, need good soil in which to grow their food. Loss of soil and reduced health of soil from current mono-cropping practice is a serious issue for the long-term survival of people on planet earth. As nutrients are depleted from the soil, the resulting food also becomes nutrient poor. Plant-based foods are also the primary drivers for clearance of the world's natural forests.

Feedlot animal farming is a dreadful way to farm, with animals often fed unnatural food, antibiotics and waste products, and I recommend that you seek grass finished meat and pastured eggs sourced from sustainable regenerative farms if you can afford to. This may be a bit more expensive, but your dollar is sending an important message that your health is important. Omega-6 levels in feedlot (cornfed) meat are 10 times higher than pastured raised meat.

If this option is not available to you, then ignore it. The nutritional benefit of grass finished meat is only slightly better than the standard US factory farm sourced meat.

Regenerative agriculture utilizing animals to re-fertilize the soil has been shown to sequester carbon from the air, generating a net reduction in carbon, meaning that this type of agriculture has an important role to play in the return to sustainability for the world. For more details on this, take a look at "https://savory.global"or "https://whiteoakpastures.com" and learn about their success in restoring desert areas to full pasture and return to sustainable food production. A huge benefit of animals is that they can eat plants grown in areas that are totally unsuitable for cropping and they have a digestive system that can process plants, such as grass, that humans cannot eat, turning these into nutritious food.

Despite what is often claimed, historically plant foods were nowhere near as available as they are today, due to lack of low temperature storage, lack of transport, short seasonal availability, and competition from diseases, animals and insects. Just look around the supermarket and consider what is in season today and could be sourced from local farms around your area, without sprays, fertilizers and cold storage. In addition, the varieties available years ago did not have anything like the same levels of sweetness, and size compared to today.

In many societies, and particularly in cooler climate areas, the only food available year around was animals and fish.

Plants don't want to be eaten and one way they fight back is by loading themselves with chemicals and anti-nutrients that are toxic to the insects and animals that eat them. There are very few human edible plants and many that we eat have to be carefully treated by cooking or component selection to avoid sickness. Despite this, a huge number of the sickness and auto immune diseases in the world are directly related to toxicity of chemicals in plants, such as gluten in wheat. All insecticides originally come from plant sources.

Plant breeding to reduce insect damage to crops often results in new varieties with even higher toxins, because these are the plants most avoided by insects.

Failure to recognize the nutrient shortages in plants has resulted in huge loss of life over the years. The epidemic of Pellagra, in the late 19th and early 20th century resulted in sickness and about 100,000 deaths in southern USA alone from eating corn (maize) that had not undergone the traditional nixtamalization treatment. This is still a problem today in southern Sahara.

Without this treatment corn lacks niacin often causing death over 4-5 years. Thiamine deficiency causing Beriberi is another example.

There are number of major edible crops that are genetically modified (GM) to be 'Roundup ready'. These include soya beans, corn, sugar beet and canola, which is a modified rapeseed. 'Roundup ready' means that the plant is modified to enable the crop to be sprayed with the herbicide, Glyphosate, and only the weeds are killed because the plants have been 'genetically modified' to resist this particular herbicide.

In addition, many crops including lentils, corn, wheat barley, and sugar cane are desiccated just before harvest, by spraying with Glyphosate to chemically dry the crop and assist harvesting. More reasons to consider avoiding products made from these plants as some research shows that Glyphosate disrupts gut bacteria in chickens, pigs and cows and is an endocrine disruptor causing tumours and breast cancer in laboratory rats. While the manufacturer may claim that animals are not effected, we have a microbiome which is apparently impacted.

Traditional treatment of plants has meant that we can get delightful taste and good nutrients from many plants and they are a complement to any diet. While bio-available nutrient levels in plants are generally lower than animal sourced food, if you decide to eat a plant-based diet, check carefully that you are getting all the nutrients you need. This is especially critical for young women who may one day have children and need to ensure that their baby is getting all the required nutrition for full baby brain development.

Does eating meat increase cancer risk? If it did, then our ancestors who ate lots of meat would have had lots of cancer, but cancer is rare in traditional societies. Doctors who treated these groups historically reported zero to very low incidence of cancer.

If you need research, check this out https://bit.ly/2nkMmx9.

If you have concerns about the death of the animals, information I have seen suggests that many more animals die due to monocropping practices of plant growers, than through regenerative agriculture. It is my belief and my own observation, that farmers who practise regenerative agriculture are very focused on the welfare of the animals in their care.

SPECIAL NOTE
FOR VEGANS

If you thought that going vegan would be easy? You just stop eating anything animal based. Well then you may be in for a health shock soon. People make different choices for their own reasons, and with some difficulty you can be vegan and still follow my health plan as outlined in this book.

To become a 'healthy' vegan you need to take a close look at the nutrition in the food you are eating. Why? You just removed a whole category of food that was supplying a massive quantity of very important nutrients to your body. You can cope for a while using stored nutrients, but your health will begin to gradually deteriorate. You will become sick more often, you will be more fatigued and will likely lose muscle mass, lose hair, and get cold more often.

What to do? Let's take a look at the nutrients.
Let's look at an example of what I am concerned about:

Consider iron from:
 100 grams of Spinach or 100 grams Beef

Starting Iron level =   Spinach 2.6 mg   Steak 2.5 mg

Iron absorption rate = Spinach 1.7%   Steak 20%
Iron absorbed =   Spinach 0.044mg Steak 0.5 mg

While the levels were similar at the start, in the end the steak provided 11 times the level of iron. In addition spinach comes packaged with oxalates which is very destructive for some people.

<u>Protein</u>. This is the master building material for your body. It builds hair, muscles, skin, connective tissue, blood, almost everything. Plant foods can provide protein, however except for some specific foods, the level is often very low and the type of protein is often not very bio-available to you. Children's growth can slow or even stop if they don't get enough protein. When planning meals you must calculate your daily protein needs at about 1-2 gram of protein for every 1 kilogram of body weight absolute minimum. If you are building muscle, pregnant or over 60 then increase this up to double the level or more.

Your body can not store protein, so if you haven't provided, it will cannibalize it from somewhere else. Few plants supplying protein have the full range of essential amino acids required by you. Without the full complement, even the amino acids supplied cannot be used. To overcome this, when planning meals, you must, match food with complementary amino acid profiles in order to ensure you are providing all 9 essential amino acids.

Many plants such as broccoli and spinach, contain good protein, however the level per calorie can be low meaning that you would have to eat a lot of it to get sufficient protein. Soy is apparently quite good, although much soy is genetically modified food (GM) and soy can drive up estrogen levels.

<u>Carbohydrates</u>. Many people who cut the animal foods, just replace these with more carbs. They become a 'carbotarian'.

Carbohydrates are sugar and supply energy, but too much energy forces your body to store the excess as body fat. Many carbs particularly processed whole grain foods like pasta, cookies, bread, cereals and bagels, have very low nutritional value, despite their high energy level. If your body is looking for nutrition or protein, it will keep you feeling hungry way after you have consumed your daily calories.

These carbs can also create a massive sugar spike, forcing your body to release lots of insulin to get the sugar out of your blood and down to the normal level of about 1 teaspoon full. I recently saw a vegan snacking on a banana wrapped in a slice of bread, wow, almost 10 teaspoons of sugar in one hit. The result is immediate fat gain.

<u>Fat</u>. Despite what you may think, eating fat does not make you fat unless you are eating it with excess carbohydrates in the same meal. Excess carbohydrates are converted to fat and stored in your fat cells that make you fat. You need lots of 'good' fat in your diet. Your brain is nearly 60% fat, your nerves are sheathed in fat, many hormones are constructed from fat, many vitamins are only fat soluble (A, D, E, K), human babies are born fat and use this fat to nourish their brain development.

Without sufficient fat you get sick very quickly. One reason for this, fat is a major component of your immune system. It is now realized that low LDL cholesterol can be an indication of an immune system under stress. You will need to plan what you eat to make sure you are getting enough fat. Avocado, coconut and olive oils are excellent but industrial seed oils (vegetable oils) are very unhealthy and should be completely avoided because they overload the body with Omega-6 and are very unstable. Did you know that the fat in human breast milk is 48% saturated fat. Saturated fat is good for you.

<u>Anti-nutrients</u>. Many plant foods contain anti-nutrients, with

the ability to lock out key vitamins and minerals from your diet by preventing your body from being able to absorb these. Carbohydrates use up large amounts of magnesium to be digested. Phytic acid which is common in seeds such as wheat, prevents the absorption of minerals such as iron, calcium, manganese, and zinc by binding to them before your body can absorb them. Oxalates found in spinach and soy inhibit the absorption of calcium. Protease inhibitors in Soy inhibit the action of enzymes pepsin and trypsin which prevents them from breaking down protein for absorption.

Vitamins B12, B6, B1, B2, niacin, and zinc are common deficiencies on a vegan diet in part to the action of these anti-nutrients.

There are a number of ways to reduce the impact of anti-nutrients, such as soaking, fermenting, cooking, sprouting with different methods working for different anti-nutrients. For example, Phytates (Phytic acid) in nuts, grains and seeds is heat resistant so sprouting works best to reduce this. If you eat a lot of corn then you must learn about the process of soaking and then cooking in an alkaline solution to make niacin available. To get the full value of any nutrient from a vegan diet, you must know all about this and apply it to each type of food you are eating.

Study the table on the next page for how to minimise the impact of anti-nutrients. For some people these have little obvious impact although they could be having a hidden impact on their long-term health. For others the impact can be immediate and maybe even life threatening.

Antinutrients

Antinutrient	Found in	Impact	Mitigation
Phytates	Grains, seeds and nuts, eg wheat.	Binds to calcium, Iron, copper and zinc.	Soaking, sprouting
Oxalates	Peanuts, almonds, potatoes, spinach, soy beans, leafy greens, many other foods	Binds to calcium, Iron, Magnesium, Potassium. May promote kidney stones.	Limited options
Lectins	Grains, legumes, peanuts	Binds to sugars and cell nuclei, affects processing, disrupts intestinal metabolism.	Soaking, boiling, pressure cooking
Salicylates	Tomatoes, night shades, mushrooms, broccoli, cauliflower, zucchini, leafy greens, tea.	Allergic reaction, itching, hives, nasal congestion, diarrhoea.	Avoid
Gluten	Grains, including corn, rice, quinoa	Triggers inflammatory reaction	Avoid
Tannins	Some vegetables, and fruit, coffee, tea, wine	Zinc & iron inhibitor	Soaking, boiling
Saponins	Grains, legumes, White potatoes, quinoa, highest in soy and haricot beans.	Weakens gut lining	Reduced by Soaking, cooking but not removed
Glucosinolates	Broccoli, cabbage, cauliflower	Affects thyroid function	Cooking reduces by 30-60%
Flavonoids	Coffee, tea, wine, onions, kale, tomatoes, berries	Inhibits mineral absorption. Act as mutagens, pro-oxidants generate free radicals, inhibit key enzymes involved in hormone metabolism.	Avoid
Protease Inhibitors	Soy beans, grains, legumes	Block absorption of some proteins	Boiling

The bottom line here is that to be a healthy vegan, you must plan your nutrition, what foods to eat and how to prepare them. If you thought it would help you lose fat, then you may be wrong. Due to the insulin spike from carbs plus other factors, many vegetarians gain fat while losing muscle mass. Vegan statistics often present well when compared with the general population, because a vegan thinks carefully about their food and tries to follow a healthy diet unlike many people who for want of education or motivation, eat very unhealthily.

On 22 August 2019, BBC news reported on an Australian couple who were charged with neglect for trying to raise a baby on a strict vegan diet without understanding the full implications. *"This child was severely malnourished, underweight and undersized and delayed as far as age-appropriate mile-stones were concerned,"* said the judge. The baby looked 3 months old despite being 19 months. Judge Sarah Huggett criticised the parents for putting her on a *"completely inadequate diet."*

A choice to not eat animals may be a case of wishful thinking. All animals eat other animals or living plants. so while you might like to live in a world where nothing has to die to support another living thing, this does not seem to be the way our world works. The death of one organism provides the building material for other organisms whether animal or plant based.

GREEN SMOOTHIE DANGER

It is possible that you are eating some toxic food but think that it is healthy? Do you eat plants that insects avoid? Maybe they know something?

You might love spinach, rhubarb, silver beet (Swiss chard), chives, parsley, soy beans, sweet potatoes, miso soup or almonds, but it is possible that by eating lots of these every day, you are loading up your body with oxalates. Particularly if eating them raw, in salads or smoothies. What are oxalates?

Oxalates are tiny needle shaped crystals and for some people, the impact on their body is highly inflammatory. Most people can handle some level of oxalates, as the kidneys can filter them, from their blood, however if the level is continuously high, then sickness could be the result. The crystal accumulation can cause generalized problems, such as poor concentration, joint stiffness, swelling, muscle pain, tendonitis, hiccups, belching, restless legs, poor sleep, kidney problems, and other inflammatory conditions. A serious outcome of high oxalates can be kidney stones (calcium oxalate).

Check out, a green smoothie cleanse causing kidney disease. (https://pubmed.ncbi.nlm.nih.gov/29203127/).

Experts assume humans can handle about 120 mg of oxalate per day, but just 1/2 cup of steamed white-stalked silver beet (Swiss Chard) has about 500 mg of oxalate and 1/2 cup of steamed red silver beet has over 900 mg of oxalate, while steamed spinach has about 700 mg per 1/2 cup. That is a lot of oxalate, but the actual levels will vary by season, soil conditions, variety and time of harvest.   Spinach is a very high oxalate food with tested levels of up to 1145 mg per 100 grams of raw wet weight. Keep in mind that this could be just one of many sources of oxalates in your meal.

For Vegans eating lots of soy and green vegetables particularly salads or green spinach smoothies and for Low Carbohydrate dieters substituting almond flour for wheat flour, this is something to be aware of.

Excess vitamin C supplementation or a lack of vitamin B6 can increase oxalates. Oxalates remove iron, calcium, magnesium and zinc from your blood, depriving you of these essential minerals.

In the ocean, mercury accumulates in the big fish as they eat the small fish with the result that the big fish can become toxic and we are advised not to eat them. Oxalates can accumulate in your body over time in exactly the same way. As you eat oxalates they can build up in various places in your body and cause localized problems as a result. If you previously ate a high oxalate diet for a number of years such as might be the case if you are vegan or a heavy consumer of spinach smoothies, then it will take some years for the level of stored oxalates to reduce. I understand that the recovery can last more than 10 years.

When your body recognizes that dietary oxalates are

significantly reduced and that it may be a good time to begin dumping stored oxalates to reduce the toxic load, an unexpected problem can arise. Apparently, the process of dumping oxalate involves extracting it from storage and putting it back into the blood for disposal by the kidneys. Unfortunately, this new high non-dietary oxalate level in the blood can be very toxic and cause problems for the liver, heart and lungs as it is disposed of. Minimizing this toxic load may require you to very slowly reduce oxalates rather than making a sudden diet change.

Sally K. Norton (https://sallyknorton.com/) is an expert on oxalates and released her book "Toxic Superfoods" in December 2022.

How can you minimize this problem right now? You can eat low or zero oxalate foods, you can balance higher oxalate foods with low or zero oxalate foods in a meal, or you can choose to eat calcium rich foods with the oxalates. The oxalates bind with the calcium in these foods which can then transport them out of the body. Examples of calcium rich foods include salmon, sardines, bone broth, and shellfish. Boiling can reduce the oxalate level by 16% to 66% depending on the food. The oxalate is discarded in the cooking water.

Low oxalate foods include meat, fish, dairy, eggs, avocado, peas, cauliflower, mushrooms, onions, and cabbage.

Many people do not seem to be impacted by oxalates and their kidneys safely flush them out in urine. Keeping this toxin under control is about knowing where it comes from and ensuring that the variety in your diet is sufficient to ensure you are not driving up oxalate levels.

BREATHING AND GUT HEALTH

While researching what to eat, I came across references to the autonomic nervous system which controls the things that happen without your conscious input, such as breathing, sweating and heartbeat. There are three divisions of the autonomic nervous system named: the Sympathetic nervous system, the Parasympathetic nervous system and the Enteric nervous system. The first two fulfil 2 opposing functions and keeping them in balance is critical to your health.

The Enteric nervous system controls the gut from when you swallow until excretion. It is able to operate independently of the brain and has been referred to as the 'Gut Brain' or '2nd Brain'. Because the gut is a tunnel from the mouth to the anus, it is actually 'outside' the body. Anything crossing the wall of the gut is actually moving from outside your body to inside your body. Nothing is truly inside us until it has crossed this barrier. Many compounds inside the gut are toxic to your body, which is why it is so important to avoid anything that makes your gut leaky.

There is a growing awareness of a solid link between brain health and your gut health. Research has a shown strong impact of persistent high glucose on the risk of dementia. Gliadin exposure, a protein found in gluten, is believed to increase permeability of the blood-brain barrier, there to protect your brain from toxic compounds and, also increase permeability of the epithelium, lining of the intestine.

Lectins in beans, grains and the night-shade family of vegetables can also exacerbate this problem in the gut through the production of the protein zonulin which is a protein discovered in 2000, that modulates the permeability of tight junctions between cells of the wall of the digestive tract. Poor gut permeability is referred to as 'leaky gut' syndrome where the body's defensive systems perceive foreign protein molecules to be a virus and an autoimmune response occurs. The body attacks itself resulting in such conditions as arthritis, type-1 diabetes, allergies, colitis and depression.

The Sympathetic nervous system, sometimes referred to as the 'fight or flight' system, is your catabolic (breaking down) system, designed to ensure that in a life threatening situation you have the maximum resources to survive. To do this, it focuses on maximising blood flow to muscles, increasing heart rate, increasing cortisol and generating adrenaline in your body. This is great when you need to escape a lion, but unfortunately many modern stress situations, or even ruminating on these situations can activate this response. It is an excellent response when needed, but sympathetic nervous system dominance, impacts health if continued for longer periods. Typical results of this include a suppressed immune system, chronic pain and inflammation.

Apparently, research with rats has shown that eating carbohydrates can activate the sympathetic nervous system as can a higher consumption of caffeine. Short shallow breathing that does not involve the diaphragm will keep the sympathetic nervous system engaged. Breathing this way tells your subconscious that danger is about and keeps stress levels and inflammation high.

The Parasympathetic nervous system, sometimes referred to as the 'rest, digest and repair' system, is your anabolic (building up) system, designed to rebuild the body and promote reproduction. It responds by providing blood for digestion, building muscle, boosting the immune system, promoting healing and maintaining fertility. It is beneficial to your health to ensure this system is frequently engaged. The parasympathetic nervous system is able to be engaged consciously by slow deep breathing utilising the diaphragm and belly. Breathing this way is telling your body that all is OK.

Apparently the only known way that you can control what signals your autonomic nervous system gets is by breathing well. This way you can help control stress and therefore how your body is responding. A slow, long exhale promotes the Parasympathetic nervous system. A recommended healthy way of breathing is longer slow breaths using the belly, where the exhale is longer than the inhale. For example: 3-4 seconds inhale and 5-7 seconds exhale. This technique can also help lower blood pressure. You can practice it regularly, in the bus, watching TV, in bed, lying in the bath etc.

My method for doing this is to breath in time with my heart beat as follows: In - 2 - 3, Out - 2 - 3 - 4 - 5 - 6. And repeat. So if your heartbeat is 72, you are slow breathing 8 times per minute.

YOUR MICROBIOME

Perhaps you are being controlled more than you realise. Ed Yong wrote a fascinating book called "I contain multitudes" in which he highlights the recent research linking your microbiome to many health conditions. Apparently, we are made up of a huge number of micro-organisms that work for us or against us depending on how we treat them. Scientists are focusing heavily on the organisms in your gut, but they are in many other parts of the body as well. I have heard it suggested that your microbiome makes up more than 60% of you.

Mary Ruddick a well respected nutritionist, says that if you have cravings, this is really the craving of your microbiome that is ensuring that you eat the food it wants. If you have sugar cravings, then your microbiome has a higher level of the bad guys.

Your microbiome is much more important than you may realise. It makes your feel good chemicals such as dopamine and serotonin, it makes vitamins, it breaks down food and much of the goodness we get from food is a result of it being consumed first by the bacteria in your microbiome. It produces B vitamins for us and can affect whether some of our genes are activated (expressed) or not. 70% of your nervous system is based in your gut lining.

There is a belief that the microbiome must be diverse to be healthy, however testing of some very healthy traditional native groups has shown that you can have low diversity and still be very healthy. Apparently, it is the quality of bacteria in your microbiome and the integrity of your gut lining that matters, whether it is diverse or not, not so much.

How do you know if your microbiome is healthy or not? One clue is whether you are craving sugars and starches. The bad bacteria in your gut including those that can cause overgrowth, thrive on sugars and starches and they will influence your brain to crave them to ensure that they get the food they want. Your good bacteria can also eat sugars and starches but have a preference for fats and protein. This suits your body perfectly because your cells also thrive on fats and protein.

If you need to clean up your microbiome, the only way to use food to do this is to starve out the bad bacteria. So a diet with no sugars or starches is required. However these bacteria can live for quite a long time, some for over 3 months. If you starve them out for many weeks, but then have a cheat day before they have died off, you will refresh them and you will have to start the whole process all over again. So that slice of pizza or spoonful of dessert at the girls night out is enough to derail your whole campaign. Only 100% adherence to the program will work. This makes it very hard for people to do. In the GAPS diet book, Dr. Natasha Campbell-McBride suggests that many months are required for effective treatment.

How will you know that you have eliminated the bad bacteria? Amongst other benefits, the cravings will be gone, you will wake up refreshed in the morning raring to go and you will feel very calm.

Unfortunately antibiotics can and usually will damage your

microbiome, so if you have taken a dose of these in recent months, you may be having to rebuild your good bacteria as well.

Some ways to help with this are:
- Minimise plant foods with oxalate toxins and lectins such as beans and spinach.
- Don't overdo the fiber and limit grains. Fiber is less important than is commonly believed.
- Eat more animal fats and totally avoid omega-6 industrial seed oils (vegetable oils).
- Get your proteins from a range of animal foods and minimise plant proteins.
- Remember that vitamins A, E, D and K2 come from animal fats.
- Avoid soy-based food and tofu.
- Get outside in the mornings to get more vitamin D and to assist with melatonin production.
- Get the sugars and starches out of your diet to stop feeding overgrowth.
- Socialise.

Intermittent fasting (IF) with a non-eating window of at least 18 hours can help with microbiome and gut lining repair as it provides an opportunity for your gut to rest and rehabilitate between the sequences of food arriving.

IF also promotes autophagy where the body can replace proteins, replace damaged cells and run a general maintenance program. An easy way to do this is to finish dinner by about 6pm and then only consume water, coffee or tea until noon the next day. See the chapter on Fasting.

LAB TEST STANDARDS

When the doctor organises lab tests, the results are compared with 'Reference Ranges' (normal levels) for each test and then the doctor is advised of any results that fall outside this range.

For example, if your HbA1c is 5.2% (33 mmol/mol) and the normal level is under 5.8%, (Under 40 mmol/mol) then all is good and sometimes the doctor will not even bother to tell you things are OK. No news is considered good news.

But an interesting question arises as to how is the reference range determined. We can't ask your body, and everyone is a little unique with some people seemingly perfectly healthy with blood test results that would be very unhealthy for others. You probably know someone or heard of someone who was a regular smoker and lived to a ripe old age, while others are sickened by second hand smoke alone.

So in order to set a reference range, results of many people are viewed over time and a level is set based on actual test results for seemingly healthy people. It is usually set at the range that 95% of the tested people fall within. Unless set by a national agency, each laboratory validates and sets their own reference ranges, due to slight differences in the testing, equipment, testing process, and differences in their test population. This must be why it is often noted that the 'normal' level will vary by laboratory.

Here is a statement from a laboratory: "*Adult reference Range values were established from wellness participants with an age mix similar to our patients*".

But what is to happen if, over time, the general results move away from the reference range? Laboratories have little choice but to 'adjust' the 'reference range' to reflect the real results they are now seeing in their patients. With only 12% of USA adults now recording as metabolically healthy, what is happening to the reference ranges for our general testing? This should be a warning to us to be aware that 'normal' may not be healthy. If your doctor is not astute about this shift in test results over time, the information you get (or don't receive) to suggest that all is good because your results are within the references ranges, may be poor.

To compound this problem, in many cases insurance, or other funders, will only authorize and cover the cost of tests where there is reasonable grounds to suspect a problem. The result is that the tests are therefore not representative of a healthy population, but are skewed towards unhealthy because only suspected unhealthy people are actually tested. If your results are in the 'normal' window, they may actually be showing that you are sick.

This from the American Center for Disease Control (CDC). In 2009, the average waist size for women in USA was 37.4 inches, in 2019 it was 38.7 inches. Any reference range (normal) for USA women will have increased by about 1.3 inches, but 'healthy' has not increased by 1.3 inches.

As an example of this, blood cholesterol reference ranges have been gradually declining, not because lower cholesterol is healthier, (it's not, read about it earlier in this book.) but because more and more people have been prescribed statins and this is gradually lowering the overall readings for cholesterol. Since we now know that higher cholesterol is correlated with lower overall death rates in people aged over 60, we have the strange situation where the doctor is seeing lower cholesterol as ideal only at lower and lower levels, while the patient would actually be healthier and have a more robust immune system with higher cholesterol levels.

So next time your doctor says that your tests have all come back 'normal', ask for a written record of the results, you may need to do your own research. I choose to keep my own record of my tests so that I can observe any progression in the results.

FIGHTING A VIRUS

I have always wondered why a virus would kill the host as this seems to limit their options to proliferate. But what if they preferred to remain a mild chronic nuisance to the host, but if the host is not very strong, they end up killing them. A living host would help them survive for a long time and to spread to many people. This model seems to fit past epidemics where many people had limited symptoms, but only small numbers died.

With this in mind, maybe the best thing you can do to minimise a virus risk, is to make your body as inhospitable to a virus as possible, which will mean it will not survive and your risk is hugely reduced.

The most important element seems to be your overall metabolic health. Those who are less metabolically healthy with underlying diseases such as Type-2 diabetes, hypertension, obesity, insulin resistance, etc are an easier target for a virus. This is because these conditions can drive up the whole-body inflammation level, which if left untreated can mask the signals telling the immune system that a virus has arrived. This unfortunately gives the virus more time to proliferate within you, before your body begins to fight back and therefore severely weakens your immune system response.

A way to tell if this applies to you is to measure your waist circumference. Then compare it to your height. If your waist measurement is more than 1/2 your height measurement, then there is a high chance you are metabolically unhealthy.

Can you change this? Surprisingly YES you can. A diet that dramatically reduces carbohydrates, and removes sugars and seed oils can begin to improve your metabolic health in as little as three weeks. A Keto or Paleo diet can help with this as can getting enough vitamin D through daily sunshine exposure. I have read of people on supplementary insulin getting off this treatment within days of such a diet change.

You can also help reduce chronic inflammation by reducing your underlying stress level and therefore your level of cortisol. Perhaps the easiest way is to improve your sleep by getting more sleep prior to midnight, and waking, after at least 8 hours, at a set time every day and getting out into the sunshine. Harder in winter of course.

Another thing that may help is to focus on removing from your body, the food that a virus can use to nourish itself. A high level of the amino acid, arginine in your body will stimulate a virus and accelerate its growth. Foods high in arginine generally come from plants and include beans, wheat grains, nuts, peanuts, chocolate, tofu, garlic, peanut butter and ginseng.

Within your body there is an arginine / lysine balance which you can influence by increasing the level of lysine containing foods. Foods high in lysine mostly come from animal sources and can suppress viruses, so include lots of red meat, pork, eggs, chicken, sardines, lamb, brewers yeast, mung bean sprouts and spirulina. Dairy products can be an excellent source of lysine.

If you are using lots of nut flours for baking, then maybe you need to eat these items with lots of dairy such as cheese or cream without sugar to keep the lysine balance high.

There are some foods that will suppress viruses by blocking the ability for a virus to attach to a cell in your body. A suggestion for this is to eat shiitake mushrooms which are relatively low cost and loaded with beta-glucans, very capable of this blocking.

Finally make sure you are getting enough zinc in your diet. This can come from oysters, beef, egg yolks, liver, dairy, lamb, sunflower seeds, pumpkin seeds and shiitake mushrooms. Apparently, zinc will attract viruses and transport them out of your body.

CHANGE IS SLOWLY HAPPENING

Recently Tracey D Brown, ex-CEO of the American Diabetics Association 'came out' and spoke about her adoption of low carb eating and the resulting partial remission of her diabetes. She anticipated being off all medication within a year. See. https://youtu.be/S6eNS7qJg38. She was also the first American Diabetes Association CEO who actually had diabetes. Why is her low carb result not being shouted from the rooftops?

From the Diabetes Canada Web site. *"Healthy low or very-low-carbohydrate diets can be considered as one healthy eating pattern for individuals living with type 1 and type 2 diabetes for weight loss, improved glycemic control, and/or to reduce the need for antihyperglycemic therapies. Individuals should consult with their health-care provider to define goals and reduce the likelihood of adverse effects."* *"Note- Canadians, with and without diabetes, who prefer to adopt a low or very low-CHO (Carb) dietary pattern, should be encouraged to consume a variety of foods recommended in Canada's Food Guide. Regular or frequent consumption of high energy foods that have limited nutritional value, and those that are high in sugar, ~~saturated fat~~, or salt, including processed foods and sugary drinks, should be discouraged."* (I added the strike thru).

https://www.canadianjournalofdiabetes.com/article/
S1499-2671(20)30097-6/fulltext

Some doctors like Dr David Unwin in the UK are now treating Type-2 diabetics by putting them on very low carbohydrate diets with intermittent fasting to reduce their insulin levels and are having amazing success with many patients achieving a full remission. This is a huge improvement from the historical, and common, practice of injecting exogenous insulin which does control the glucose but, it raises insulin levels, which drives weight gain and other complications for the patient. It is also a much lower cost solution with many patients no longer needing the insulin injections.

I look forward to the day that government or state health agencies prioritize this low carb treatment to drastically reduce their health budgets.

EARLY NUTRITION PIONEERS

How fascinating. My reviews of research into nutrition, health and medicine has uncovered some interesting information from the 19th and early 20th century with some really interesting pioneers. You may have heard of some of these people, but many will not be known outside a very small and interested group. Again, as covered in this book, most of them are trained doctors who, because of what they observed in their patients or themselves, decided to do their own research and came up with their own treatment guidelines.

William Banting, (1796-1878) an undertaker, published one of the most famous early reports of his experience following a low calorie diet in 1863, which emphasized restriction of bread, butter, milk, sugar, beer, and potatoes with portion controlled meat for breakfast and dinner which allowed him to lose 50 pounds in one year. His pamphlet titled "A letter on Corpulence" is available on the internet, was translated into multiple languages and sold widely for decades.

Dr. James Salisbury, (1823-1905), was an American physician who undertook food experiments on paid volunteers and on his pigs. He has the Salisbury Steak named after him. One of his main approaches to dietary research was to feed his pigs or volunteers a single substance over time, and to record the results. He would often autopsy his pigs following experiments to establish what impact the diet had had. For his human subjects if they got to ill he would stop the testing. Interestingly to restore the health of his human experimental subjects he always reversed their condition and returned them to full health by feeding then just beef and water. He documented his experiments in his book "The Relation of Alimentation and Disease" published in 1888 and available from the University of Leeds as an e-book.

Western A. Price (1870-1948) was a Canadian Dentist who explored the relation between health, diet and dental health, by travelling the world and documenting the diets and health conditions of native groups. He sought out groups who were mainly eating their traditional diet in order to compare this with "modern" diets. He discovered that ancestral eating groups consuming their traditional diets had little dental decay and were generally in good health. He found that within a generation of exposure to "modern" diets with refined grains, most of the native groups began to show negative health signs. He identified that smaller jaws and impacted teeth, child birth difficulties and many other conditions he observed appeared to be directly related to a move away from traditional diets. I would recommend visiting the website https:// westonaprice.org for more information.

Dr. Vilhjalmur Stefansson (1879-1962) was an explorer who lived with the Canadian Inuit for a number of years. He published at least 4 books including "My Life With The Eskimo", "The fat of the Land" and "Not by Bread Alone". In 1928 after returning from a long period in the Arctic he was challenged to prove his claims about surviving on a meat-only diet. A colleague and himself checked into the Belleview hospital where they were fed a fatty meat-only diet for a year. Various specialists gathered to "witness" his expected development of scurvy but were disappointed when he never succumbed to this sickness. Apparently fresh meat contains a small amount of vitamin C plus a very low carbohydrate diet has a much lower need for this vitamin.

At the completion of one year, both of the test subjects were examined and pronounced fully healthy. In fact, his colleague was in better health than at the beginning of the year long trial. The all-meat diet was a resounding success providing sufficient fat was left on the meat. Without the fat, people can suffer from "rabbit starvation" which is described in my book.

Otto Warburg, (1883-1970) a German cancer researcher who worked in Nazi Germany is described in Sam Apples excellent book titled "Ravenous". For his discovery that cancer uses glycolysis for synthesizing ATP from Glucose, he was awarded the Nobel prize in 1931. Here was the proof that cancer uses sugar for its metabolism and that depriving it of sugar by limiting dietary glucose or minimising insulin or both, will weaken cancer and possibly kill it. Unfortunately, because he was a Jew, but was not treated like other Jews by Hitler, a number of people felt he was a Nazi sympathizer. It is suggested by Sam Apple that he was spared due to Hitlers absolute obsession with Cancer and as a result, supported the research.

Dr. Walter Yellowlees (1917-2014) was a Scottish doctor based in Aberfeldy in the Scottish Highlands. He attended medical school from 1936 and served in the army medical corps in the Second World War. He has written a book titled "The Doctor in the Wilderness", where he sets out his observations of health and diet of the years following WW2, up to his retirement. While some of his observations have been proven to be wrong, such as the cause of stomach ulcers, (Australian Doctors proved that these were the result of the bacteria Hector Pylori). His view that many serious modern diseases are the direct result of a diet that is too heavy in sugar, white flour and seed oils is close to the mark. He laments the state of medicine there the "obvious" impact of these substances is routinely ignored in health and nutrition advice.

Surgeon Captain T.L. Cleave, (1906-1983) a doctor working with the Hunza People in Northern India and a senior surgeon in the Royal Navy until his retirement in 1962 has produced a book about diet and nutrition. His final book titled "The Saccharine Disease" published in 1974 sets out his belief, from his role of Director of Medical Research for the Institute of British Naval Medicine, that many diseases are the result of excess consumption of white flour and sugar, and that a return to less highly refined food with the resulting reduction in carbohydrates from refined sugar and refined flour is needed.

As a result of his work, he was elected to the fellowship of the Royal College of Physicians and the Harben Gold Medal in 1979 by the Royal Institute of Public Health and Hygiene for outstanding discoveries in the promotion of public health. He was also awarded the Gilbert Blane Medal for work in promoting health in the Royal Navy. Despite this recognition, his work is largely forgotten and certainly not applied to nutrition guidance for health.

Walter. L. Voegtlin MD, F.R.C.P. (1904-1975) Has written a book titled "The Stone Age Diet" published in 1975. Born in 1931, he was an American gastroenterologist and pioneer of the Paleolithic diet. His well written analysis of the history of Western nutrition and how it came to be so messed up (even by 1975) highlights the need to eat meat for good health and complete nutrition.

Dr Wolfgang Lutz, (1913-2010) an Austrian doctor who for a number of years worked in an isolated community in the European Alps. He successfully treated a number of his patients with low carb diets (zero bread) and in 1967 he published a book titled "Life without Bread". Unfortunately for us, a number of European doctors nutrition research was largely ignored following the war and was sidelined perhaps because of the German WWII defeat.

Dr. Robert Atkins (1930-2003) was an American physician and cardiologist best known for the Alkins Diet. He was not a researcher but a practising physician and wrote a number of popular books based on his experience of treating patients with low carbohydrate diets. Thousands of people found his books helpful for losing weight and improving their health. His departure from the accepted standard of care generated many critics and following his death from a fall he was subjected to may "theories" that his diet was the cause of his death. To the delight of his critics, these wild theories seem to be regularly repeated. It is disappointing to find the focus frequently is on these theories rather than the positive results he achieved with so many people.

In 1982, researchers Bistrian and Blackburn, at the Harvard Medical School published results of a low carbohydrate diet called "A Protein Sparing Modified Fast" where calories were limited to 650 - 800 per day. On this diet, 668 patients lost significant weight with about half losing around 40 pounds or more over 17 weeks. There were no side effects. However, at the time it was widely believed that a low carbohydrate diet with higher saturated fat was unhealthy and therefore they discontinued the work. We now know that carbohydrates are not necessary as the human body can synthesize glucose from fat, plus we have also learned that higher saturated fat consumption does not correlate with higher mortality.

It is very clear from these pioneers that some of their work has been ignored but is now coming back into vogue. Much of the information in this book is supported by these early pioneers which is unsurprising as it posits a return to an earlier time and style of diet before the advent of ultra-processed food, big pharmaceutical companies and the domination of a few powerful food companies.

GETTING STARTED

If you decide that this healthy life choice is for you, then I offer the following tips. Your initial focus should be on reducing your insulin level and returning your body to insulin sensitivity. Prepare to find your refrigerator full and your pantry with less in it, because you are eating more real food. Real food spoils quickly if left out of the refrigerator.

This is NOT medical advice. I am not a health professional; this is merely documenting what I have come to believe from my personal journey reviewing research plus my personal results. Prior to making any changes to your diet or lifestyle, you should seek professional medical advice from a registered health professional.

What 'Carbohydrate level' should you be aiming to eat daily, remembering that very low carbs is not a problem for your body? The Dr. Atkins approach is to target about 20 grams of carbohydrates daily and then as you begin to get close to your goal weight, add back a few grams of carbs each week until your weight stabilizes. In the 1960's Austrian Dr. Wolfgang Lutz identified that 72 grams of carbs was the sweet spot for health maintenance. Maybe keep away from Omega-6 seed oils forever, but find a target carbohydrate level that suits your body.

My experience is that calorie, glucose and ketone measurements are not necessary. Make life simple, just avoid the heavy carbohydrate laden food such as sugar, potatoes, rice, grains, cereals, bread, pasta, donuts, industrial seed oils and products made from these.

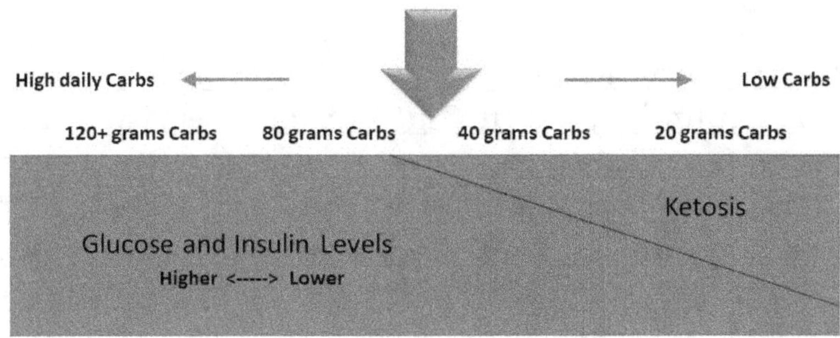

The switch from a 'sugar-burner' to a 'fat-burner' is not instant and will take a few days minimum, maybe weeks to get adjusted and can involve mild side effects. For many people the carbohydrate restriction needs to be applied gradually over time to give the body room to adjust to this major change.

If you have been eating a very high carbohydrate diet with upwards of 200-300 grams of carbs per day, then you are probably better to switch more gradually as your body could struggle with such a big change. In this case, maybe first drop your carbs level to about 100 grams per day for about 2 months to make sure there is no discomfort, replacing the other carbs with protein and fat.

Maybe start by reducing sugar, then starchy vegetables, then grains over a few weeks. To achieve a reduced insulin level could take a while, particularly if you are currently insulin resistant, because your body is accustomed to having to produce excess insulin in order to achieve the required hormone signalling. An adjustment period is often needed to overcome this and regain insulin sensitivity.

For some people getting into ketosis can take months, but keep in mind that the objective is not to get into ketosis, this is just an additional benefit. The real objective is to lower glucose and therefore insulin levels in the blood to improve your overall health.

<u>If you are currently prescribed any medication especially external insulin, then you must have supervision by your medical professional to ensure care with any change process. Your body's sugar balance is critical and errors here can result in very serious problems. Perhaps warn your doctor that some diabetics on insulin have had to reduce external insulin levels within days of this change.</u>

Although a Keto or LCHF diet is not an 'eat fat' diet, make sure you eat sufficient good quality fat and protein so that you are not feeling hungry. The reduction in carbohydrates must be replaced by an increase in protein and fat. Remember that eating fat does not make you fat when carbs are kept low. See the comments about my dietary fat level in the 'My Results' chapter.

The good news is that a blood ketone level of more than 0.4 mmol/L results in a suppressed appetite so you rarely get hungry between meals. The aim is not to eat a lot less calories, or you may kick your body into starvation mode and your metabolism will slow. So, keep up your calories, and do not snack between meals. Remember your goal is to keep insulin levels low. Eating the required level of fat is quite difficult at first as it goes against all past conditioning. If there was a golden rule it would be, eat when you are hungry, stop when you are full.

Plan your meals because there is generally more preparation required due to less off-the-shelf items available. An easy help to meal planning is to cook larger meals each dinner time and refrigerate the excess for the next day's breakfast or lunch. This helps, as you are adjusting to a higher level of home cooked food.

Keeping up hydration is critical and you may need to supplement salt, magnesium and possibly potassium as the reduction in carbohydrates increases the water loss and this can lead to loss of these essential minerals. I have found that I need to take about 1/2 teaspoon of salt in warm water each morning.

Adjusting to a reduced level of fiber in your gut can take a little time and you may find that you settle into a new regular pattern where bowel movements are less frequent with less volume than you were used to. Mild constipation can be an indication of insufficient fat in the diet, or insufficient fluids, so drink plenty of water, add salt, add more butter to the vegetables and olive oil to the salads. Eat all the fat on meat and buy the cheapest and fattiest ground beef (mince). In my experience your body will soon settle down to a new normal and you get to love the taste.

Some people believe that humans are required to have 1 bowel movement each day or they have constipation. I have not found this and frequently have days without any movement. There is no problem, I am just using up more nutrients in my food, so leaving less waste for excretion. I effortlessly catch up on the following days.

The release of stored fat may release toxins and hormones that were originally stored in the fat. This can create some temporary hormone swings and unexpected body responses as the liver deals with this load. The good news is that apparently pollutants in the body can decrease by about 15% after fat loss.

For traveling food or easy lunches, I suggest some hard-boiled eggs, avocado, cheese, salami slices, ham slices, canned tuna or sardines, some nuts, cold sausages, and some crackers. A green salad with some vinegar and olive oil dressing is also a good option. You could still choose a hamburger but chuck the bun and avoid sugary sauces. Read labels to avoid fish canned in seed oils.

Be aware that for many people, there exists a very real addiction to processed food (carbs) that is super tough to break. Apparently, this is one reason we often hear about people who tried keto, but then claim that it did not work for them. It can take some people up to 8 weeks to get adapted to the change. Ensuring that friends and family are aware and are supportive could help. For these people, it seems that almost complete carb abstinence for a long initial period is the only way to success, with any small 'treats' triggering a wholesale return to 'full-on' carbohydrate consumption. I guess this is the same for an alcoholic, full abstinence is necessary.

A thought: You never hear it suggested that an alcholic could have a cheat day!

Your first thoughts are likely to be focused on all the foods you seem to be losing and how will you replace them in your diet. Over time you will adapt to the change of diet so that some foods that seemed indispensable at the start eventually become unimportant. For example, I used to eat cereals every morning and loved them, but now I don't ever feel like breakfast. I don't miss spreads because we no longer eat foods that need them. I loved Mac and cheese, but we have switched to cauliflower cheese bake, (see in Recipes) yum.

I eat more crackers than ever and have to bake them nearly every week to keep up supplies because store bought crackers are often full of unhealthy seed oils and sugar.

We no longer buy much fruit, milk and bread, but we buy many more vegetables, cream, meat, avocados and 72%+ chocolate. We also waste much less food as all the left-overs get eaten up over the next few days.

If you find that you are not getting the results you expect, or you have reached a plateau, then it is possible that too many carbohydrates are creeping back into your diet from:

- Nuts or nut butters

- Sugar in berries, chocolate or sugar substitutes,

- Starches from those in-ground vegetables like carrots and potato.

- Check out the ingredients in anything you buy for hidden sugars.

- You may need to tighten up on your diet discipline, at least initially in order to progress, because everyone's personal 'carbohydrate threshold' is different.

Remember that in order to have your body consume stored fat, you must be eating a little less than your body needs each day, so watch those meal sizes.

Stress and poor sleep can also impact results as they trigger cortisol which stimulates glucose and insulin release.

It will be useful to recall the discussion about fiber at the start of this book. You will be eating less fiber and this means a much smaller urge to poop. Look out for that smaller urge and respond to it to avoid small hard stools. You will get adjusted over time.

Your body gets used to what it is asked to do and often learns to anticipate. This shows up when you condition yourself with training such as running or exercise. If you have been eating a full on diet of heavy carbohydrates with cereals or toast for breakfast for years, it is quite likely that your body is adapted to dumping a load of insulin into the digestive system in readiness for that rush of glucose it has to deal with. When you make such a big dietary change by reducing carbohydrates like this, that adaption may take a little time to change. So take it slowly and expect a few bumps at the beginning.

GUIDANCE

To help you on your way, here are a few thoughts that might assist with the transition:

1. Plan your eating. This means deciding a time and place for each meal and also deciding when during each day, you are not going to be eating.

2. Take a good look at the meal plan, plan your shopping and visualize yourself following through with each meal.

3. Think about the size of the food on the plate, not too small that you will imagine yourself as being hungry soon afterwards, but not so big that you will be stuffed. Remember that it can take some time for your body to recognize the "I am full" message.

4. Start to focus your new knowledge on those foods that are unhealthy for you, particularly those old friends that you have now learned are killing your health goals. Imagine what damage they can be doing to you. If you do feel a little smug about this new knowledge then revel in it.

5. Think about the period between your meals when you will not be eating, and plan what your will be doing in that time, maybe exercising, working, sleeping, socializing, etc.

6. Look at the meal plans and think about what might become

your new favorites. Plan to learn how to prepare these well, so that they look good on the plate and also taste delicious.

My web site https://www.takebackyrhealth.com contains free sample meal plans plus other resources.

7.   Take a look in the pantry and refrigerator and clear out those temptations that you have agreed are not going with you on your health journey. If you are a baker, you might want to think about giving away those recipe books that are not part of your new food health journey.

8.   Imagine how you will respond when tempted with foods that are not part of your journey so that when a waitress offers you the bread basket, you can politely and immediately turn it down without any temptation. Think about how you will respond to friends or family that don't have this knowledge of good nutrition and may not be very supportive.

9.   Take another look at the foods that you have selected as treats and ensure that you have some of these available for when you need a little boost.

10. As you become more used to these meal choices, you will be able to visualize yourself selecting the right food choices. Think first about the protein on your plate. Is it sufficient to satisfy your protein appetite? Only after getting this right, should you think about the other parts of the meal.

11. As each day is won and you have managed to stick to the plan, congratulate yourself for your achievement. This is a change that for some can be as difficult as giving up smoking or alcohol.

12. Make some notes in your food diary about what you liked, how you feel and what is working for you. This will become valuable input to help guide you on your new lifestyle journey and it will reinforce, the choices you made today.

For many people there exists a selection of up to 20-30 core meals that are the go-to meals for much of their eating. A great move is to start to plan what you will include in a new selection. Once these are defined, meal planning will become as easy as riding a bicycle. Some may not change; some old favorites will be consigned to the unhealthy bin. Maybe you can share new recipes with friends and learn together which ones you want to repeat regularly. Enjoy the journey.

HERE ARE MY EATING GUIDELINES

1. Minimise Carbohydrates, think NO GPS, don't eat Grains, Potatoes or Sugars. (Corn, wheat and rice are grains). So limit bread, pasta, bagels, cookies, pastry, pancakes, cereals, honey, muffins, rice cakes, fries, buns, cakes, etc., unless these are made with nut flours and butter or coconut oil.

2. Avoid Omega-6 polyunsaturated seed oils. (Canola, corn oil, soya oil, safflower oil, rice bran oil, sunflower oil, grape seed oil, cotton seed, margarines, shortening, etc.).

3. For cooking, use fats normally solid at room temperature including saturated fat such as butter, coconut oil, lard and use tallow for deep frying.

4. For liquid oils use fruit oils, olive oil (cold pressed), avocado oil, or warmed coconut oil. An olive oil / vinegar mix makes an excellent salad dressing.

5. Eat fish, meat, eggs, nuts, dairy (If you can) including cheese, cream and low sugar / full fat Greek yoghurt but no milk.

6. Avoid ultra-processed food, only eat real food. Food with a

nutrition label is most often ultra-processed.

7. Eat plenty of vegetables, especially those grown above ground as they generally have lower carbs.

8. Avoid anything labelled as 'low fat', because to make it taste good, manufacturers often add extra sugar.

9. Adapt to a less sweet diet by avoiding sugar and artificial sweeteners.

10. For fruit, try to eat only small servings of fresh berries, strawberries, blueberries, raspberries, mostly avoiding bananas, grapes, apples, plums, peaches, etc. except for the occasional treat. Try to limit larger fruits to 1 a day and eat the whole fruit. No juicing.

11. Have small amounts of dark (>72%) chocolate as treats. Check nutrition panels as some dark chocolates still have a high carb level.

12. For medication, avoid NSAIDS such as Aspirin, Ibuprofen.

13. Drink pure water, tea, green tea, hibiscus tea, coffee, and avoid milk, fruit juices, soda and alcohol.

14. Salt to taste, more is better than too little salt.

15. If you are dining out, try to avoid deep fried food.

16. If you are having a few carbs with a meal, try to eat them at the end of the meal.

17. Make sure you keep up your protein level, particularly if you are an older woman. The 0.8 grams per Kilogram guideline is just a minimum survival level. You should be eating about 2x

this level and up to 3.0 grams of protein per kilogram of lean body weight. I am assured that this is not dangerous for your kidneys provided you have no kidney disease.

A meal with meat or fish plus lots of vegetables followed a little later, by a coffee or green tea and a small piece of dark chocolate, is an excellent choice.

The more I learn about what is going into ultra processed food, the more resolve I have to avoid eating it. At this point I have full control over what is going into my body. I make my choices, and my money will relay my choice to food providers.

MISTAKES YOU CAN MAKE

I have learned that there are some key mistakes that I can make on this 'lifestyle', so I will document them here so you can benefit as well:

- Eating too little fat. I need to ensure I am eating plenty of fat, as my fat phobia from years of 'wrong education' makes this difficult. Ensure it is always good fats, avoiding seed oils and margarines.

- Too much fat can also be a problem. If you are eating tons of fat, your body will never need to utilise body fat for energy, meaning that you won't lose any body fat. So take it easy with the bullet proof coffees. For myself, I never have these or MCT oil. I have not needed them.

- Eating enough protein. Don't fear protein. The talk about it overpowering kidneys is apparently overstated and not supported by medical trials. I personally need about 100 grams of protein daily to maintain my body. Because I am older and exercise regularly, I may need more than some people. Higher protein levels can also lower your personal weight set point, which is the level your body is trying to keep you at. This may be a benefit to you. Regularly over eating will raise this setpoint.

- Eating the wrong fats. I need to ensure my dietary fats are saturated fat, monounsaturated fats and Omega-3 polyunsaturated fats, minimising the Omega-6 seed oils. Although Omega-6 oils are essential, the level needed is miniscule and is likely to be provided in what you eat.

- Not enough salt. The Keto diet is a diuretic and lowers salt, plus I am avoiding salt laden processed foods so I need to ensure my salt level stays up. I drink 1/2 a litre of warm water with 1/2 teaspoon of salt every morning. For me, it has zero impact on my blood pressure. Higher salt intake is critical if you suffer migraines.

- Too much fasting ie: longer than 24 hours. It is important to avoid having my body feel that there is a famine, because if it does, it will begin slowing my metabolism. I need to ensure I am eating well.

- Dehydration. Because the low carb diet reduces water retention, it is easier to get dehydrated. If your stools become hard, read the section on fiber, eat more fat, and drink a little more water each day but not while eating as it can dilute digestive juices. During the first few weeks of the diet change I worried about this as I missed my previous regular bowel movements. Over time this stabilised and I learned that I had no reason to be concerned. Due to the smaller stools, I sometimes miss a day but it does not seem to matter. Monitor the color of your urine, clearer is better.

- Avoid eating processed foods. Read labels carefully until you get proficient. Watch out for vegetable oils, soy, canola, corn oil, sugars, MSG (e621), etc.

- Carefully read nutrition labels. Note the serving size and number of servings on the nutrition label. Sometimes this can hide higher levels of the bad stuff.

- I suggest you don't get too hung up on whether the meat and eggs you eat are pasture finished or not. Many peoples in the world would be healthier with some animal food and cannot afford the premium price of grass finished. We should recognise this and campaign for the animal sourced food foremost before worrying too much about the source. If you can afford it then support the local farmers who are seeking to improve the food chain but don't denigrate others who may not be able to.

- Overdoing sugar substitutes. These can also spike insulin and may make lowering the overall level of sweetness hard for you to manage.

- Too many nuts and seeds. While good to eat, do some have relatively high levels of carbohydrates.

DINING OUT

Ordering in restaurants is tricky and I have learned some things:

- Unhealthy seed oils are likely to be used in all cooking and also added to food. Ask for cooking in butter.

- Most restaurants are willing to substitute, for example replace potato with mushrooms.

- Fish often comes battered, crumbed or grilled. If you don't ask it is usually battered. Grilled is healthiest.

- A 'Big Breakfast' can make an excellent base for building a meal. Ask for it to be cooked in butter.

- A roast meat meal can also be a good start for building a healthy meal as there is plenty of protein. Just hold the potatoes.

- A good healthy ploy when eating out is to double the protein in the food. For example, asking for double meat in a burger (no bun), double eggs or double bacon. This ensures that you are getting sufficient protein but might cost extra.

- Chinese food is tricky because of the abundance of sauces with sugar and soy. However, they do some great meat based dishes and seem to be happy to hold the rice.

- Some restaurants are better left to their usual customers. Be willing to leave. For example: a pizza restaurant, although you could just eat the toppings.

- Even when ordered right, often the process fails, so carefully check orders.   Some waitresses are keto aware and can make great suggestions.

- Carry your own salad dressing if you want to be sure. I like an olive oil, vinegar mix. You can usually ask for the sauce on the side.

- Sometimes you just have to order and then leave what you don't want on the plate. However, this can result in a small meal.

- Telling them what you don't want allows them to top up the meal size with items you do want, after all they want the meal to look good as it comes out to the table.

- Restaurants serving older customers often have good options including organ meat, such as liver and kidney which are super full of nutrients. Liver is perhaps the most nutrient dense food available, but I wouldnt eat it too often, once a week is enough.

- When all else fails, the occasional higher carbohydrate meal will actually help you maintain metabolic flexibility. Remember that stress causes cortisol release which increases glucose, so don't stress about a few extra carbs.

- For your overall health, the single most important thing is to avoid the 8 industrial seed oils (called Vegetable Oils).
  Canola

Corn oil
Cotton seed oil
Grape seed oil
Rice Bran oil
Safflower oil
Soy bean oil
Sunflower oil

STARTING GRADUALLY

I made the switch cold turkey and found it to be relatively easy, but for some this won't be the case. Here is a suggested step by step approach:

Week 1,
Check in with your medical advisor. There are a lot of very dedicated doctors and nutritionists out there that want to make a difference. Some through lack of up-to-date knowledge will be very hesitant. Others are keen to learn and may already be prescribing low-carb diets to some patients. Seek out these doctors if you can. Get out the tape measure and measure the before waist and take some 'before' photos.

Week 2,
Eliminate all sugar and products with added sugar. Read labels for 'other' sugars. If the name of the ingredient ends in -ose, then it is likely a name for sugar. Think about sugar substitutes, or better, reduce sweetness over the whole diet. Finish up the fruit and give away the sweet treats to unsuspecting others. Check sauce labels such as barbecue sauce, as they are often packed full of sugar. There is a tendency to rush to artificial sweeteners to

maintain that sweet taste, but I suggest lowering the sugar level in stages and avoiding the artificials.

Week 3,
Remove Industrial seed oils from the pantry replacing with good oils. Cook with butter, avocado oil, coconut oil, animal fats, adding extra virgin olive oil to salads.

Week 4,
Eliminate processed food from the diet. No more cereals or packaged meals. Get a couple of good Keto recipe books or check out websites like https://www.dietdoctor.com. You might switch to having eggs for breakfast, maybe with bacon or mushrooms, yum. Breakfast does not have to be cereal based. It never was before packaged cereals arrived.

Week 5,
Replace all wheat based products, including bread, pasta, bagels, chips, cakes, etc. Explore bread and cracker replacements, see the recipes at the end of the book and the notes on travelling food.

Week 6,
Replace the other grain products including rice, quinoa, oats, barley, etc. Clean out the pantry, and stock the refrigerator with cheeses, meats, eggs, etc. Make sure you are keeping up your protein level.

Week 7,
Identify replacements for potatoes and corn and identify new vegetable staples, cauliflower, broccoli, asparagus, spinach, kale, avocado, etc. Find recipes that will take you forward with snacks, lunches and breakfasts. Try new things and identify new family favourites.
Get out the tape measure and compare with those early measurements.

MY RESULTS

Does it work for me? YES, Absolutely. Weight down 11kgs (24 lbs.) over 15 months. Waist measurement down 4 inches, LDL (bad) cholesterol down, HDL (good) cholesterol level up, Triglycerides level way down, HbA1c level down, Blood pressure down, from 2 medications to zero. Strength and muscle mass maintained. I am now 72 years old and comfortably do 15 chin ups, 40 push ups, single leg squats, and can comfortably run 5Km each morning. My waist measurement is less than 1/2 my height measurement and I now comfortably fit clothing that I wore when I was 18 years old.

I have an old pair of monogrammed white overalls I wore when I worked part time in a bread factory as an 18 year old to fund university studies. I now comfortably wear them occasionally when painting.

In 2017 my triglyceride to HDL ratio was 2.48, today it is down to 0.80. Ideal is less than 1.5. my BMI is now 22.5.

I weigh myself each morning, and check my blood pressure about twice a week. Blood tests each 6 months. Nothing else gets measured regularly.

My Weight, Kgs in the First Year

Dropped about 10 Kgs (22 Lbs)
Over the first 12 months.
Then it began to level off as if
my body now realised that I had
reached a healthy weight.
Note the bump at Xmas.

This graph is my record
in the Apple Health App.

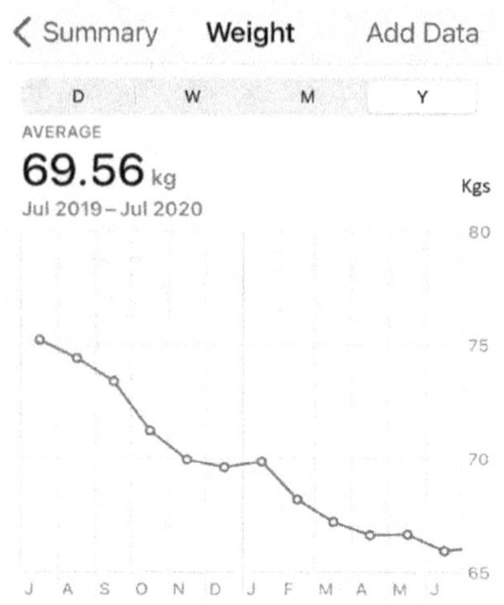

After 12 months, I analysed 8 weeks of my diet in great detail. This is what I found I averaged per day:

Protein   115 grams, calories (25%)
Fat   129 grams   calories (63%)
Carbohydrate   57 grams   calories (12%)
(My protein level is 1.7 grams per Kilogram weight)

Satisfaction levels are massive. I have no hunger. I feel like I have found the secret to good health.

IN THE KITCHEN

Someone asked me what staples we had in our kitchen, so I took a look and here is the list I created:

Almond flour
Coconut flour
Green banana flour, (Only used as a fresh fish coating)
Ground Psyllium Husk
Sesame seeds
Flax seed or ground flax seed
Baking powder

Pink Himalayan salt
Iodized salt (make sure you are getting iodine)
White salt flakes in grinder
Black pepper in grinder
Oregano
Onion powder
Garlic powder

Apple cider vinegar
Balsamic vinegar (low sugar)
Mayonnaise (low sugar, low Omega 6)
Tartare sauce (low sugar, low Omega-6)
Butter

Camembert cheese or Brie
Cottage cheese
Cream (full)
Cream cheese
Eggs
Hard cheese (Cheddar)
Edam or Mild Cheese
Mozzarella cheese
Parmesan cheese
Brie
Sour cream
Thickened or double cream
Unsweetened full fat Greek yoghurt
Unsweetened tartare sauce (ideally)

Coconut oil
Avocado oil
Olive oil, (extra virgin, best quality)
Tallow (for deep frying)
Lemon juice
Lime juice

Bacon
Mince or Ground Beef (fatty)
Pork sausages or Pork Mince
Steak
Other meats.

Sardines in spring water
Tuna in olive oil
Tomato paste, (low sugar)

Almonds (Tamari)
Macadamia nuts

Dark chocolate, > 72%

Stevia, Erythritol or Monk fruit sweetener (sparingly)

Vegetables:

Broccoli
Brussel sprouts (occasional)
Cabbage
Capsicums
Carrots (used sparingly)
Cauliflower (or Frozen cauliflower rice)
Celery
Green beans
Lettuce
Onions, Brown, red and spring
Parsley
Peas (used occasionally)
Salad mix, Rocket
Silver beet, Chard
Spinach
Tomatoes
Zucchini for Zoodles

Avocado
Blueberries (occasional)
Raspberries
Strawberries

I know some items here are not strictly Keto, but that is OK for me as my macros are where I want them.

RECIPES

It is not my intention to turn this into a recipe book. There are plenty of these out there and they are backed by clever chefs with huge experience. However here are some basic recipes that I believe helped my wife and I to make the transition to a Keto / Low Carb diet.

Crackers.
Cauliflower Bake.
Bread rolls.
Toast.
Blueberry Ice-cream.
One Dish Beef and Cabbage.
Blueberry muffins.
Pizza.

Crackers

I searched the supermarket aisles, reading the nutrition information of many crackers, looking for something that could be used as a base for a snack or quick lunch. All crackers seem to be full of industrial seed oils, sugars and wheat flour so I went looking for a recipe instead and here it is. You can have these topped with cheese, tuna, salami, egg, sardines, dip or a huge number of other options to replace a meal or for an easy snack.

George's Crackers

Makes about 50 small crackers.

Ingredients:

- 6 Tbsp of ground flax seed.
- Unground flax seed passes directly through the gut without digestion.
- Ground flax seed must be stored airtight in a refrigerator as it goes rancid quickly.
- 2 tsp of salt. (+ Extra grinding salt for topping).
- 4 cups of almond flour.
- 12 or 13 Tbsp of water.
- 2 Tbsp of fine grated parmesan cheese (optional)

Method:

Grind flaxseeds in coffee grinder, if required.
Mix dry ingredients in a bowl, then mix in fine grated cheese if desired
Add water and hand mix until the dry mix turns into dough.

Place dough between baking paper layers and press or roll out to about 3mm (1/8 inch) or less.

I divide my dough between multiple mixes to suit the available oven tray sizes

Keep thickness very even to prevent the edges from burning during baking

Remove top baking paper layer.

Use a pizza cutter to cut cracker size squares. I make mine about 30mm (1-1/2 inch) squares.

Wetting the pizza cutter helps prevent the dough from sticking to the cutter wheel.

Don't separate the crackers.

Grind a fine layer of flaked salt over the dough and gently pat down by hand.

At this point you could experiment with other toppings such as sesame seeds or (my favourite) black pepper.

Bake in oven at 150 deg C (300 F) for 45-50 minutes. Adjust baking time until they are golden brown.

When done, immediately slide off the baking paper onto a wire rack to air cool and crisp up.

Store once completely cool.

They store for a couple of weeks.

Cauliflower Bake Recipe

This recipe came from the waitress in a local restaurant. Adjust quantities to suit yourself.

Identify baking dish (about 12" x 7" about 1-1/2" deep)
Fill baking dish with florets of fresh cauliflower
Mix bacon & onion dried soup mix powder with some grated cheese
Sprinkle over the cauliflower florets
Pour over 1 cup full cream
Bake at 180 C (350 F) for 45-50 minutes

You may need to cover to prevent burnt edges.

This is so tasty and often lasts for 2-3 meals.

Keto Bread Rolls Recipe

There are a lot of very similar bread recipes available and this one is quick and easy without being too eggy. Makes about 8 small rolls.

Ingredients:

150 gram Almond flour.
40 gram Psyllium husk powder.
2-1/2 tsp baking powder.
1 tsp salt.
2 tsp cider vinegar.
2 eggs.
1 cup boiling water

Method:

Heat water.
Mix all dry ingredients in a bowl.
Fold in cider vinegar and beaten eggs.
Add boiling water while hand mixing.
Form into rolls using hands moistened with olive oil.
Place on baking paper on baking tray.
Bake for 50 minutes at 175 C (350 F).

Can be split, toasted and buttered, or fill and eat These store well in the freezer. You can form the buns larger and get 4 hamburger buns.

Toast Recipe

To make this we cook a tray of bread about the thickness of 2 slices of toast. Then when cooked, cut into toast size squares and then divide these into toast thickness slices by splitting each square into 2 layers.

Makes about 16 small toast slices.

Ingredients:

5 cups almond flour
3 tsp baking powder
2 eggs mixed with 1/2 cup cream beaten together.
Add in some grated cheese.
Black chia seeds (optional)

Method:

Mix together, then spread out in
baking paper lined sponge roll tin or similar
about as thick as 2 slices of toast.
Cook for about 15 minutes at 200 deg C (400 deg F)
Add cheese on top. (optional)

When cool, split into toast as above. Instead of splitting into toast, it can also be left whole and eaten as scones.

Blueberry Ice-Cream

This is a small recipe for one.

Into a cup put a handful of whole frozen blueberries.
Pour in liquid full cream up to the same level as the blueberries.
Leave for a few minutes for the cream to freeze.
With a teaspoon, dig out frozen cream with blueberries and eat.

Makes a great after dinner or small dessert treat.

One Dish Beef And Cabbage

I really like the crunchy cabbage and oiliness of this dish. Can make 4 meals.

Ingredients:

500 grams ground beef or beef mince.
    (can use pork mince if you wish)
About 350+ grams of chopped up cabbage, I like it chunky, but my wife likes it chopped fine.
(Include more chopped up stalk to keep it crunchy, or omit to have it softer).
1 large onion chopped fine.
1 powdered soup mix (Bacon and Onion) mixed in 1 cup of cold water.
1 tsp of curry powder, or more if you love curry.
2 Tbsp coconut oil or butter
Salt and pepper to taste.

Method:

Chop cabbage and onion and put aside.
Heat oil in large pan and brown the ground beef, breaking up any big lumps of meat.
When meat is browned, add in chopped onion and cabbage, cover if possible to keep steam in.
Mix the soup powder and water then add into the pan.
Sprinkle in the curry powder and turn to mix in.
Keep turning the food to ensure it cooks evenly and keep the temperature up to ensure plenty of steam.
(Add 1/2 cup of water if it seems a bit dry.)
Add salt and pepper to taste.
Keep turning and now remove the lid to allow the final steam to

escape.
When it is all cooked and the food is just starting to brown on
the pan bottom, it is done.
Serve and eat.

Yum

Makes great left overs for the next days lunch.

Blueberry Muffins

These muffins are very low carb and are great for a snack when you need something with that coffee or green tea. Makes 6 small muffins.

Ingredients:

1 cup almond flour
1/4 cup monk fruit sweetener
1 tsp baking powder
30 gram melted butter
2 Tbsp full cream
1 tsp vanilla essence
2 large eggs (whisked)
1/4 cup of blueberries

Method:

Prepare a muffin tin with 6 muffin liners.
Preheat oven.
In a suitable bowl, mix all the dry ingredients.
When mixed, add the melted butter, vanilla and eggs. Stir until mixed well.
Add blueberries and gently fold into the mix.
Divide the mix into the 6 muffin liners, trying to get an equal amount of blueberries into each.
Bake at 180 deg C (360 deg F) for 20 minutes or until the tops are golden.
Cool on wire rack before eating.

Pizza

Pizza is easy and very much liked by us, and so when switching to Low-carb (Keto) we went looking for a good replacement pizza recipe. Some are very cauliflower dominant, while others are almost totally cheese, although some of these taste very good. After trying out a number of pizza recipes with varying results, we came across this tasty recipe. Preparation is very easy and fast.

Makes 4 medium servings with added salad.

Pizza Base Ingredients:
185 grams (6-1/2 oz) grated mozzarella cheese
40 grams (1-1/2 oz) cream-cheese
1 tsp Onion or Garlic powder
100 grams (4oz) almond flour
1 egg size 7 (Large)
Salt and pepper to taste

Toppings:
50 grams (2oz) grated Parmesan Cheese
Select your own toppings, such as tomato, scallions, bacon, ham, pineapple.

Method:
Preheat oven to 220° C, or 425° F
Allow egg to warm up to room temperature.
Select and oil a suitable flat dish or tray, or you can use baking paper (best).
Soften Mozzarella and Cream-cheese in a bowl in the microwave, stir together then cook for about 30 seconds on high.
Add the Onion powder, Almond flour, Egg and a little salt and

pepper.
Mix well, then tip onto baking paper on tray and
    press out evenly until it is about 3mm (1/8 inch) thick.
Top with your choice of toppings then add a layer of grated Parmesan Cheese.
Bake until the everything looks tasty, about 20+ minutes.
Serve hot.

Enjoy.

FURTHER LEARNING

If you are interested in the history of nutrition and the influence of corporations and ideology on our diet, take an hour to listen to Belinda Fettke on YouTube here: https://youtu.be/NEFvoyTMxVg

I have now read well over 200 books plus YouTube video's, and podcasts. Here is a very small selection of some of the books I have read which you may also like to read.

- Why We Get Fat, by Gary Taubes.
- The Big Fat Surprise, by Nina Teicholz.
- Keto, A womens guide, by Tasha Metcalf (2019).
- Eat Like The Animals, by David Raubenheimer & Stephen J. Simpson (2020)
- Lies My Doctor Told Me, by Ken D. Berry, MD, FAAFP.
- A Fat Lot Of Good, by Dr. Peter Brukner OAM, (Dr. for the Australian Cricket Team).
- What the Fat, How to Live The Ultimate Low-Carb Healthy Fat Lifestyle, by Schofield, Zinn and Roger (2015).   (*This is a New Zealand based book*)
- The Case For Keto, by Gary Taubes (2020).
- Keto-tarian, by Dr. Will Cole (2018).
- The Carnivore Code, by Dr. Paul Saladino MD (2020).
- The Obesity Code, by Jason Fung MD.
- Keto, by Maria and Craig Emmerich (2018)

- End Your Carb Confusion, by Eric C. Westman MD.
- The Clot Thickens, by Dr. Malcolm Kendrick

There are many more, and what is really fascinating is that many are written by doctors who became sick following standard nutrition guidelines. They realized that something was wrong, did their own research, changed their diets and cured themselves with food as medicine. Having improved their own health, they were so motivated that they wrote their experience into books for others.

On Twitter, follow Dr. David Unwin, @lowcarbGP to follow the success he is having reversing type 2 diabetes.

An excellent resource for recipes and guidance, is the web site: "https://www.dietdoctor.com".
Also check out the book and movie 'Sacred Cow' released in late 2020.

'Take back your health' by using your food as medicine, George Elder (2020). www.takebackyrhealth.com

ABOUT THE AUTHOR

George Elder

George Elder lives in New Zealand with his wife and following his discovery of how wrong his understanding of nutrition was, set out to research the truth. He has graduated with a diploma in nutrition from the Nutrition Institute and has spent a huge amount of time reading and researching nutrition. 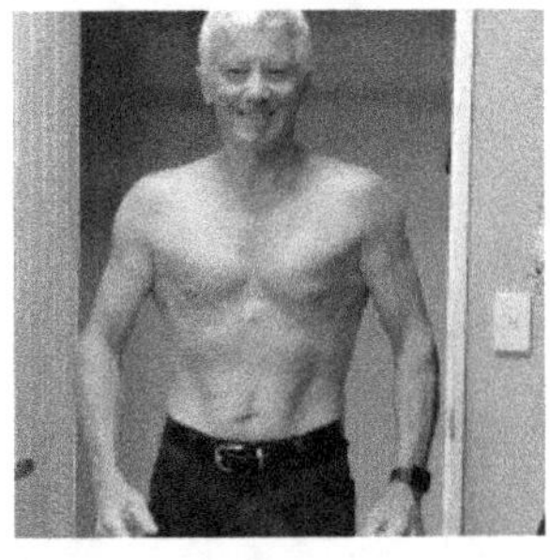

He has two grown up children and three grandchildren. He has an MBA from Canterbury University and has spent most of his working life in Information Technology and Manufacturing roles. He is a keen outdoors person having run a number of marathons, and enjoys hiking, kayaking, fishing and cycling.

As a result of his nutrition learning, his own health has improved and he is active in helping others to learn how to take back their health. George maintains a blog at www.takebackyrhealth.com